T0339696

Narrating the Heritage of Psychiatry

Narratives and Mental Health

VOLUME 1

The titles published in this series are listed at *brill.com/nmh*

Narrating the Heritage of Psychiatry

Edited by

Elisabeth Punzi
Christoph Singer
Cornelia Wächter

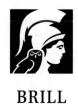

BRILL

LEIDEN | BOSTON

Cover illustration: Created by text-to-image AI, Midjourney bot.

Library of Congress Cataloging-in-Publication Data

Names: Punzi, Elisabeth, editor. | Singer, Christoph, 1982- editor. |
    Wächter, Cornelia, editor.
Title: Narrating the heritage of psychiatry / edited by Elisabeth Punzi,
    Christoph Singer, Cornelia Wächter,
Other titles: Narratives and mental health ; v. 1. 2667-0518
Description: Leiden ; Boston : Brill, [2025] | Series: Narratives and
    mental health ; volume 1 | Includes bibliographical references and
    index. | Identifiers: LCCN 2024027463 (print) | LCCN 2024027464 (ebook) | ISBN
    9789004519831 (hardback ; alk. paper) | ISBN 9789004519848 (ebook)
Subjects: MESH: Psychiatry--history | Mental Disorders--history | Narrative
    Medicine--methods | Mentally Ill Persons--history | Hospitals,
    Psychiatric--history
Classification: LCC RC454 (print) | LCC RC454 (ebook) | NLM WM 11.1 |
    DDC 616.89--dc23/eng/20240731
LC record available at https://lccn.loc.gov/2024027463
LC ebook record available at https://lccn.loc.gov/2024027464

Typeface for the Latin, Greek, and Cyrillic scripts: "Brill". See and download: brill.com/brill-typeface.

ISSN 2588-7823
ISBN 978-90-04-51983-1 (hardback)
ISBN 978-90-04-51984-8 (e-book)
DOI 10.1163/9789004519848

Contents

Acknowledgements

First of all, we would like to extend our heartfelt gratitude to all contributors to this edition. We would also like to thank the anonymous reviewers for their constructive feedback.

We are, moreover, very grateful for the financial support of the Centre for Critical Heritage Studies (CCHS) at the University of Gothenburg, Sweden.

For her careful proofreading and editorial work, we would like to offer a special thanks to Elisabeth Frank (University of Innsbruck).

Figures and Tables

Figures

Tables

Notes on Contributors

Dr Nicole Baur
is a health geographer with a strong interest in heritage studies, particularly mental health heritage. She completed her PhD at the University of Heidelberg in Germany in 2005 and has since been working at several Russell Group universities in England and Scotland. She has been researching the Devon County Mental Hospital since 2007 and has authored and co-authored articles on her research in international journals and made several contributions to books. Dr Baur also regularly organises public events to engage local communities with their mental health heritage.

Dr Verusca Calabria
is an Oral Historian and a Senior Lecturer in Health and Social Care, School of Social Sciences, Nottingham Trent University (UK). Calabria's research sits at the intersection of the history and heritage of mental healthcare. Currently, she is the Principal Investigator of a National Lottery Heritage Fund project entitle "Fifty Years of Middle Street Resource Centre: The Heritage of Wellbeing in the Community". She co-founded and co-convenes the NTU Oral History Network and is a trustee of the Oral History Society, UK.

Elena Demke
grew up in East Germany, after involvement in the 1989 citizen movement she studied history, and a Rhodes scholarship took her to Oxford. She worked as a historian for the Berlin commissioner for the Stasi-files, 1999–2018, specializing in visual history of the Berlin Wall, the didactics of political education and history politics in twentieth century Germany. Personal experience stimulated her interest in survivor-led alternatives to psychiatry, also in terms of epistemologies. Alongside her job, she studied psychology at the FernUniversität in Hagen, and got involved in peer counselling at the Verein zum Schutz vor psychiatrischer Gewalt e.V. Since 2018, she has conducted research on "meanings of objects in the context of extreme mental distress, madness and psychiatric intervention", which is a Mad Studies contribution to an interdisciplinary research group working on crises and meanings of things in various times and cultures, funded by the German ministry of education and research.

Rob Ellis
is a Reader in History at the University of Huddersfield, UK. He has published widely on the histories of mental ill-health and learning disability and has worked in partnership to co-produce projects that have emphasised their contemporary relevance.

Tomke Hinrichs

studied History, French and Educational Sciences at the University of Bremen and Rouen (France) and history at the Technical University of Dresden. During and after her studies she worked as research assistant at the "Institut für Sächsische Geschichte und Volkskunde" Dresden and as scientific staff-member at the State Museum of Archaeology Chemnitz, where she also is the curator of the exhibition about Salman Schocken. For the exhibition, she spent a short time in Israel for research purposes. Since 2013 she is working on her PhD-Project: "A subject as an object of psychiatry? – (Re-)Subjectivation in psychiatric space based on 'psychiatrised' writers of pamphlets ('Irrenbroschüren') around 1900". She has been a full-time teacher of history and French since 2017.

Dr Rob Light

is an independent scholar. He has published work as an oral historian and worked in AHRC-funded public engagement projects examining histories of mental health care.

Helena Lindbom

holds a bachelor's degree in social anthropology and is a retired journalist. She has for periods of her life experienced overwhelming psychological distress and has been in out- and inpatient psychiatric units for several decades. She was a patient in those days when heavy medications with devastating effects were used, medications that are no longer permitted, and she senses that this part of the past should be neither forgotten nor superficially excused or overlooked. Helena has worked with creative writing groups for elderly citizens and is interested in heritage and history, in literature and reading, and in spending time in nature.

Hedvig Mårdh

PhD Art History, senior lecturer in Cultural Studies at Karlstad University. Mårdh is an art historian researching public art, scenography and museum practice. In two research projects funded by The Swedish National Heritage Board and Formas she has been studying art and creative processes in former psychiatric hospitals.

Veikko Pelto-Piri

is a social worker and doctor of medicine. He works in the psychiatric administration, mainly with method support in the prevention of coercion and violence. His research focuses on coercion, violence, ethics and prevention. Veikko has previous experience of working in institutions both for people with intellectual disability and mental illness, he has also former experience of psychiatric care as a patient.

Elisabeth Punzi

is a licensed psychologist, specialist in clinical psychology, specialist in neuropsychology, PhD and associate professor at the Department of social work, Gothenburg university, Sweden where she is also director of doctoral studies. She also works for the Center for Critical Heritage Studies, Gothenburg University, where she directs the work with heritage and wellbeing. She teaches courses in mental health and research methodology and has a research interest in the heritage of psychiatry, Mad studies, and in the meaning of creative expressions and places.

Geoffrey Reaume

is Associate Professor in Critical Disability Studies at York University in Toronto, Canada. He earned his PhD in History (1997) at the University of Toronto and his work was published as a book, *Remembrance of Patients Past: Patient Life at the Toronto Hospital for the Insane, 1870–1940* (OUP, 2000). His study was made into a play performed by psychiatric survivors in Toronto from 1998–2000. Reaume is a co-founder of the Psychiatric Survivor Archives of Toronto and co-editor with Brenda LeFrancois and Robert Menzies of "Mad Matters: A Critical Reader in Canadian Mad Studies" (CSPI, 2013). He created the first university credit course in Mad People's History which he has been teaching since 2000.

Cecilia Rodéhn

holds a PhD in Museum Studies from the University of KwaZulu-Natal (South Africa) and works as a senior lecturer at the Centre for Gender Research, Uppsala University (Sweden). Rodéhn is the project manager of the project *From Psychiatric Hospital to Condominium – Urban Development and Cultural Heritage* (2020–2023) funded by FORMAS, the Swedish Research Council for Sustainable Development. She has previously managed the project Ulleråker – disability and cultural heritage funded by the Swedish National Heritage Board (2016–2019). Rodéhn's research explores representations of Mad people in cultural heritage.

Marta Wandt

is a visual artist based in Gothenburg, Sweden. She has studied at several art schools, including Hovedskous konstskola [Hoveskous art school]. She has own experiences of mental distress and of psychiatry. She says: "Through painting,

I recognize myself and my feelings and I become recognized by others. To find connection, both within oneself and in one's life. It gives a sense of restitution."

Jenny Wetterling

is active in RSMH (National Association for Social and Mental Health, Sweden) and has worked with different developing projects in the psychiatric field for many years, she has former experience of psychiatric care as a patient. The last years Jenny has been working mainly with implementation of Peer Support and The Suicide helpline. She is a registered nurse working in acute paediatric care.

Introduction

Elisabeth Punzi, Christoph Singer and Cornelia Wächter

Ever since its birth as a discipline, psychiatry has been imbued with con-
troversies. Over the past decades, biomedical perspectives have become
domineering, framing psychiatry as a science disconnected from contextual
and cultural values and practices (e.g. Horwitz 2021; Puras and Gooding 2019).
The mainstream narrative, dominated by psychiatrists, conceives of the development of psychiatry in terms of linear progress. It considers current practices
to be humane, effective and scientific, whereas earlier forms of psychiatric
care are deemed inhumane and unscientific. Such narratives of progress can
not only be found within psychiatry – here defined as the research, teaching and practices of applied psychiatry – but also in popular discourses and
practices. A case in point are old psychiatric buildings serving as memorials
of 'dark heritage', displaying gruesome treatment methods of the past, such
as lobotomy tools, electroconvulsive therapy devices, or the straightjacket as
"the most paradigmatic image of confinement" (Majerus 2017, 264). As Laurajane Smith observes, heritage can serve to "[frame] a set of cultural practices
that are concerned with utilising the past for creating cultural meaning for the
present" (2015, 459). Former psychiatric hospitals turned into heritage sites frequently not only cater to sensationalism (Rodéhn 2020, 206) and "consumerist
interest in 'dark sites' of death and disaster" (Moran 2016, 137); they also serve
to present current practices as more humane by comparison and may thus
contribute to the occlusion of ongoing injustice. They exemplify that "the discourses that frame our understanding of heritage are a performance in which
the meaning of the past is continuously negotiated in the context of the needs
of the present" (Gentry and Smith 2019, 1149).

According to John Jameson, "[i]n most countries, the authorised heritage
discourse (AHD) has dominated interpretation at managed sites reflecting
an elitist narrative, displaying and requiring technical knowledge and insight
to be comprehended" (2019, 4). In the words of Jeroen Rodenberg and Pieter
Wagenaar, "[c]ertain narratives are articulated and become dominant, resulting in objects and cultural traditions being authorised as heritage, at the cost
of others" (2018, 3). This is significant in that "inclusion in a society's symbolic
landscape means access to resources and opportunities" (*ibid.*, 5). Metaphori-
cally speaking, certain authorised heritage discourses may result in a kind of
discursive confinement by excluding perspectives, voices and stakeholders.
Consequently, the present volume asks: Whose narratives become neglected

© KONINKLIJKE BRILL BV, LEIDEN, 2025 | DOI:10.1163/9789004519848_002

or silenced? Whose narratives are perceived as important to preserve? Who is given the authority to speak 'truth' about the history and heritage of psychiatry and mental health care? And how are these heritage-discourses being constructed, which immaterial and material form of heritage do they employ to narrate the heritage of psychiatry? In line with these questions a variety of articles in this collection approach narratives and discourses in the Foucauldian sense as 'counter-discourses' and discuss the often hidden, forgotten and repressed voices therein.

Michel Foucault famously emphasised that knowledge and power are inextricably entwined, and he was among the first scholars to question dominant narratives of psychiatric progress. Presumably, the best-known example is his unmasking of Pinel's 'liberation' of the inmates of the asylum at Bicêtre as a replacement of one form of confinement by another. Rather than being constrained by chains, the person under treatment was now induced to confine themselves by strictly regulating their behaviour according to moral standards, while the physical chains continued to loom in the background, in case this regulation should fail. Such normalising pressures live on, beyond deinstitutionalisation, in the neoliberal imperative of self-care. Moreover, such pressures subsist in the form of assertive outreach teams, who medicate people in their homes. Thereby, the community has become an arena for pharmaceuticalisation, with the constant possibility and threat of being incarcerated if one does not comply with suggested interventions. Additionally, users/survivors of mental health services and, more generally, people suffering mental distress, are frequently subject to marginalisation and oppression; they are more frequently affected by poverty and various, often intersecting forms of disempowerment, and their perspectives are often discredited on the grounds of their diagnoses (see Beresford 2022, 1, 3).

In recent years, considerable effort has been made to achieve the inclusion of diverse perspectives and voices as part of a wider trend in critical approaches to heritage. Rebecca Madgin and James Lesh, among others, point to "the growth of people-centred conservation [that] is providing new ways of thinking about historic places, the reasons why they matter to individuals and collectives and how this knowledge can influence the protection of the past" (2021, 1). For instance, due to the work of psychiatric survivors and their collaborations with stakeholders, memorial plaques have been established by a wall of the former Toronto Hospital for the Insane, in order to draw attention to the fact that this wall had been constructed by means of the forced labour of inmates in the late nineteenth century (Reaume 2016). Moreover, as Dolly MacKinnon and Catharine Coleborne point out, there is now a diverse body of collections outside the AHD aiming to memorialise psychiatry in its previous formations (2011, 6). What unites most of these collections, neverthe-less, is "their use in writing the evolutionary history of psychiatry, where the past represents a 'horror' that contrasts with the more enlightened practices of the present" (2011, 6). Even art, as historian Dorothea von Hantelmann observes, may serve to promote such narratives. She points to the fact that "[t]he exhibition in its canonical nineteenth-century formation – and the museum itself – [...] marks time into a series of stages that comprises a linear path of evolution [...]" (2010, 10).

The significance given to the mentioned collections, artworks, and the per-sonal narratives associated with them, points to a growing awareness of the relevance of intangible heritage as part of what Rodney Harrison describes as the "discursive turn" in heritage studies (2013, 9). Immaterial heritage not only includes the narratives attached to material objects, the ways in which they are rendered meaningful, but it might also refer to, for example, oral histories, as exemplified by the chapter "Narratives of De-Institutionalisation: Patient and Community Responses to Mental Health Closures in England" in this volume. Harrison observes that, "[w]hile the discursive turn has been impor-tant in drawing attention to the knowledge/power effects of heritage and its processes of identification, exhibition and management, it has also tended to deprivilege the significant affective qualities of material things and the influences the material traces of the past have on people in the contempo-rary world" (*ibid.*). It is thus significant to consider the affective dimensions of remembering, or "highlighting the affective relationships that we have with our past" (Tolia-Kelly et al. 2017, 1) – not only in light of the impact of psychi-atric treatment on those subjected to it but also regarding the fact that users/survivors of psychiatry are frequently the targets of circulating negative affects. To borrow the words of Divya Praful Tolia-Kelly et al., the contributions to this volume demonstrate that "feeling the past through embodied presencing of geological/environmental space-time is core to understanding identity, differ-ence and alterity at heritage sites", and they regard memory "as an affective tool for the co-constitution of embodied, political narratives" (2017, 3).

A prominent section of the book is dedicated to activist challenges to dominant practices of memorialisation; thus, for instance, achieving the pres-ervation of a wall built by means of the forced labour of patients and endowing it with memorial places. The volume discusses pamphlets as counter-discursive endeavours to destigmatise users of psychiatry and to challenge normativ-ity; it relates the endeavours by user organisations in Sweden to probe and counter-narrate the heritage of psychiatry as part of a wider quest to promote the replacement of paternalistic psychiatric practices by more user-centred and inclusive approaches, which includes learning from earlier user groups; it also disentangles psychiatric heritage from the material heritage of madness and mad people.

In spite of what the cited examples of memorialisation might suggest, in general, there is a tendency to disregard the heritage of psychiatry and mental health care both in material and immaterial terms, and few former psychiatric buildings have actually been preserved as material heritage. John Pendlebury, Yi-Wen Wang and Andrew Lang include former psychiatric hospitals in what they term "uncomfortable heritage" (2018, 212) and observe that "[t]ypically, in creating a new use for a building with an unsavoury past, there will be a process through which the building's representation and meaning changes" (*ibid.*, 213). Graham Moon et al. identify four major trends regarding former psychiatric architecture: *retention*, where the buildings are repurposed for administrative healthcare; *dereliction*; *transinstitutionalisation*, where, for example, the architectural structures of confinement are redeployed for punitive imprisonment; *residential use*, which is especially prominent in urban locations, sometimes even forming 'gated communities', thus repurposing structures built for confinement to now keep 'intruders' out (2015, 6–7). As Paul Ricœur has famously argued, "[i]t is [...] the selective function of the narrative that opens to manipulation the opportunity and the means of a clever strategy, consisting from the outset in a strategy of forgetting as much as in a strategy of remembering" (2006, 85). Not only does an overemphasis on detrimental effects of psychiatric treatments of the past on the mental health and well-being of those subjected to it serve to occlude the continuing presence of such 'traces of a dark past in the present'; narratives of the heritage of psychiatry also tend to overlook – or strategically forget – empathetic and holistic perspective and approaches of the past, which had underlined the importance of well-being, meaning-making and belonging. These tend to be excluded from the dominant narrative.

The neglect of considering and preserving the narratives of, for instance, the users/survivors and those challenging the dominant discourse at any given point in time, might be expressive of a sense of guilt for the oppressive practices that have taken and are still taking place. It might also be connected to ideas of progress, as though we live in an era of scientific breakthroughs with no need to either look back or look sideways, or to efforts to deflect attention from the overwhelming suffering experienced by clients. Acknowledgement of psychiatry's immaterial and material heritage holds the potential to broaden the perspectives on its history as well as on current and future practices. We need to consider which parts of psychiatry's heritage should be acknowledged and preserved. What current practices are remnants of oppressive historical practices and perspectives? We also need to consider how questions of heritage might provide possibilities to formulate criticism and provide alternatives, for example through activism, user movements, visual art, handicraft, or creative writing, and also how creative expressions contribute to well-being and recovery and to scholarly and clinical insight.

For those reasons, the present volume presents counter-narratives, including community narratives, to the dominant discursive formations on the heritage of psychiatry, valorising the narratives of those who have so far largely remained unheard. It subscribes to Brian D. Orthel's claim that "[h]eritage work, heritage practices, and humanity will benefit if valid and viable connections exist between history, heritage, and health" (2021, 4). Accordingly, *Narrating the Heritage of Psychiatry* echoes Dolly MacKinnon's and Catharine Coleborne's emphasis of the "importance of the role of twentieth-century psychiatric communities in the preservation, interpretation and representation of the history of mental health through the practices of collecting" (2013, 4).

While the museum and other heritage sites may, by and large, cater to narratives of progress, the position of the observer, of course, also enters the equation. As Erica Ander et al. emphasise, "[w]hen [people] have a museum encounter, whether in everyday life or in a healthcare institution, the impact the museum resource will have on their well-being should be affected by their physical environment, the social situation and their personal levels of interest, motivation and current well-being and health" (2013, 230). What is more, art, like literature, can "give voice and image to the ones who are silenced and invisible" (Vinitsky 2017, 161). Besides the academic articles, *Narrating the Heritage of Psychiatry* is therefore framed and interspaced by artworks of a psychiatry user: Marta Wandt.

1 The Chapters

The first article "Unsettling the Past: Creating a Multi-Vocal Heritage of Exminster Hospital through Co-Production and Performance" sets out to challenge and counteract the institutional influence of authorised heritage discourses (AHD) when it comes to processes of understanding, preserving, communicating and transmitting heritage. Nicole Baur focuses particularly on heritage discourses concerning Exminster Hospital, in Exeter, UK, and highlights how changes in the theorisation but also the conceptualisation of heritage can be used to expand participation in heritage discourses and to create a multi-vocal narrative, including the voices of former clients and employees of this particular hospital. Baur illustrates not only how omnipresent the hospital still is in the village but how different artefacts and narratives complement the author-ised heritage discourse.

In their article "Lillhagen Is Still Elsewhere: Approaching a Dismantled Mental Hospital", Elisabeth Punzi and Helena Lindbom demonstrate the idea of a multi-vocal heritage by way of the examples presented here. They stress the importance of approaching and understanding dismantled mental hospitals with respect to embodied memories and sensations. Their article gives voice to and brings into dialogue two perspectives, one professional and one personal, namely that of a clinical psychologist, researcher and lecturer in social work and of someone, who has a background as a journalist and former psychiatric patient at some of the now dismantled mental hospitals in Sweden. These two perspec-tives and approaches not only imbue the spaces at hand with different narratives but also contribute to a multi-vocal and multi-perspectival creation of heritage.

Rob Ellis and Rob Light similarly seek to expand the voices and perspec-tives on the heritage discourses surrounding a specific hospital. Their research explores the oral histories collected at the Storthes Hall Mental Hospital in Northern England. In their article "Narratives of De-Institutionalisation: Patient and Community Responses to Mental Health Closures in England", Ellis and Light collect and give voice to the hopes and fears of patients and the wider communities as the hospital was closed down in the 1980s. By means of a meta-analysis, this chapter brings into dialogue broader questions asked at the time, with the local communities' responses to these processes of de-institutionalisation providing a counter-narrative to the often-privileged voices of psychiatrists.

The subsequent article by Veikko Pelto-Piri and Jenny Wetterling is also focused on the effects of de-institutionalisation and narratives surrounding these processes. In their study "From Paternalism to Social Inclusion? User Organizations' Narratives of Psychiatric Services in Sweden", Pelto-Piri and Wetterling explore the impact of influential user organisations and their perspec-tives and narratives on these processes. The methodological approach to these narratives is inspired by art history and focuses on transformation as well as a desire for and a lack thereof. In addition to narratives by user organisations, the article also outlines the history of these organisations and their interactions with other (political) stakeholders and their forms of activism and political activity.

The question of activism in relation to constructing and remembering the heritage of mental hospital is equally central to the article "Plaques, Politics and Preservation: Publicly Memorialising Mad People's Labour History". Geoffrey Reaume's case study offers a diachronic account of how different stakeholders were involved in, interacted with each other during activists' attempts to pre-serve the boundary-walls at the former Toronto Asylum for the Insane and how this history was coopeted by psychiatrists and some historians. The importance of the wall lies in the fact that these walls were built by former patients themselves and are as such an expression of the realities of this institution. Reaume particularly highlights that by publicly memorialising these walls, patient-labour is reframed as exploitation rather than therapy.

Cecilia Rodéhn is similarly interested in analysing how the heritage of a particular institution, here Ulleråker, a former psychiatric hospital located in the town of Uppsala in South-Eastern Sweden, extends beyond the walls of this asylum itself. In the study "Street Names and the Narration of Madness in a Post-Asylum Landscape", Rodéhn explores the cultural history of the asylum by tracing streets named after poems by the Swedish poet Gustaf Fröding, a former patient at the hospital, and the political processes and decisions that lead to their respective naming. Rodéhn connects these heritage discourses with 'mad readings' to question and to deconstruct the sanist discourses embedded in the naming processes and to simultaneously highlight the subversive notions embedded in these street names.

Tomke Hinrich's article "Normality Narrative in the Context of the Lunatic Rights Movement" is equally concerned with often opposing discourses between practitioners and clients. Hinrich's focus, however, is not concerned with processes of de-institutionalisation but the very opposite: namely the beginnings of psychiatry and its implementation and institutionalisation in Germany at the turn of the nineteenth century. The article is interested in people who became the subjects of psychiatric treatment against their will, particularly in cases in the context of the lunatic rights movement of the 1980s onward. Hinrich's heritage archive consists of pamphlets written by these patients in which they shared their experiences made in asylums. This article highlights how these pamphlets can be understood not only as personal expressions but as counternarratives that challenge the notion of normalcy/illness.

Hedvig Mårdh's study of the integration of art and artistic practices in former mental health care institutions, entitled "'the small point through which time passes' – Art and Artistic Practices in Former Mental Healthcare Institutions", similarly explores the notions of normalcy/illness especially the discursive associations made between mental health and artistic creativity. Mårdh explores the effects of including artistic practices and particularly contemporary art in sites with a complex history such as former psychiatric hospitals. As with other studies in this volume, the Mårdh focuses on specific and localised case-studies, here the redevelopment of Ulleråker, a former psychiatric hospital in Sweden. By looking at photographic practices in abandoned sites, as well as pre-study work by Camille Norment and public artwork by Lies-Marie Hoffmann heritage-management is discussed in relation to the concept of 'third-time'.

Elena Demke's article "Re-Assembling the Social in So-called 'Mental Illness'? Reflections on the Uses of Material Culture in the Historiography of Psychiatry and in Mad Studies" is indebted to the material turn and is interested in materiality in experiences of mental crises, madness and recovery outside their psychiatric definitions. To do so, the Demke looks at how materiality has been addressed by Mad Studies. She then proceeds to discuss the findings from a project that relies on object-elicited interviewing and (ex)user/survivor-control with the intention to create a "digital museum of madness and recovery/discovery."

The final chapter of this volume, Verusca Calabria's "'There was an awful lot that was good and that was necessary': The Hidden Heritage of the Old State Mental Hospitals", focuses on the memories of mental health service users and workers from the second half of the twentieth century. Calabria examines oral histories in order to draw on the often-positive aspects of hospitalisation and the care that was received or provided, in contrast to the usually negative connotations in the discourse of mental institutions. The study emphasises that there is no unified narrative in the legacy of residential psychiatric care, and a sense of nostalgia, both in ex-patients and staff, is presented.

References

Ander, Erica, Linda Thomson, Guy Noble, Anne Lanceley, Usha Menon, and Helen Chatterjee. 2013. "Heritage, Health and Well-Being: Assessing the Impact of a Heritage Focused Intervention on Health and Well-Being". *International Journal of Heritage Studies* 19 (3): 229–42. https://doi.org/10.1080/13527258.2011.651740.

Beresford, Peter. 2022. "Introduction." In *The Routledge International Handbook of Mad Studies*, edited by Peter Beresford and Jasna Russo, 1–16. *Routledge International Handbooks*. New York, NY: Routledge.

Coleborne, Catharine, and Dolly MacKinnon. 2011. "Seeing and Not Seeing Psychiatry." In *Exhibiting Madness in Museums: Remembering Psychiatry Through Collections and Display*, edited by Catharine Coleborne and Dolly MacKinnon, 1–13. Abingdon, Oxon: Routledge.

Gentry, Kynan, and Laurajane Smith. 2019. "Critical Heritage Studies and the Legacies of the Late-Twentieth Century Heritage Canon." *International Journal of Heritage Studies* 25 (11): 1148–68. https://doi.org/10.1080/13527258.2019.1570964.

Horwitz, Allan. 2021. *DSM. A History of Psychiatry's Bible*. Baltimore: John Hopkins University Press.

Jameson, John H. 2019. "Introduction: The Critical Junctures of Archaeology, Heritage, and Communities." In *Transforming Heritage Practice in the 21st Century:*

Contributions from Community Archaeology, edited by John H. Jameson and Musteață Sergiu, 1–12. Cham: Springer.

Madgin, Rebecca, and James Lesh. 2021. "Exploring Emotional Attachments to Historic Places: Bridging Concept, Practice and Method." In *People-Centred Methodologies for Heritage Conservation: Exploring Emotional Attachments to Historic Urban Places*, edited by Rebecca Madgin and James Lesh, 1–15. London: Routledge.

Majerus, Benoît. 2017. "The Straightjacket, the Bed, and the Pill." In *The Routledge History of Madness and Mental Health*, edited by Greg Eghigian, 263–76. London; New York: Routledge.

Moon, Graham, et al. 2015. *The Afterlives of the Psychiatric Asylum: Recycling Concepts, Sites and Memories*. Farnham: Ashgate.

Pendlebury, John, Yi-Wen Wang, and Andrew Law. 2018. "Re-Using 'Uncomfortable Heritage': The Case of the 1933 Building, Shanghai." *International Journal of Heritage Studies* 24 (3): 211–29. https://doi.org/10.1080/13527258.2017.1362580.

Puras, Dainius, and Piers Gooding. 2019. "Mental Health and Human Rights in the 21st Century." *World Psychiatry* 18 (1), 42–43.

Reaume, Geoffrey. 2016. "A Wall's Heritage: Making Mad People's History Public." *Public Disability History* 1, 20.

Ricœur, Paul. 2005. *Memory, History, Forgetting*. 5. Chicago: University of Chicago Press.

Rodéhn, Cecilia. 2020. "Emotions in the Museum of Medicine: An Investigation of How Museum Educators Employ Emotions and what these Emotions Do." *International Journal of Heritage Studies* 26: 201–213.

Rodenberg, Jeroen, and Pieter Wagenaar. 2018. "Cultural Contestation: Heritage, Identity and the Role of Government." In *Cultural Contestation: Heritage, Identity and the Role of Government*, edited by Jeroen Rodenberg and Pieter Wagenaar, 1st ed. 2018, 1–10. *Palgrave Studies in Cultural Heritage and Conflict*. Cham: Springer International Publishing.

Smith, Laurajane. 2015. "Theorizing Museum and Heritage Visiting." In *The International Handbooks of Museum Studies*, edited by Andrea Witcomb and Kyle Message, 459–484. West Sussex, UK: Wiley-Blackwell.

Tolia-Kelly, Divya Praful, Emma Waterton, and Steve Watson. 2017. "Introduction: Heritage, Affect and Emotion." In *Heritage, Affect and Emotion: Politics, Practices and Infrastructures*, edited by Divya Praful Tolia-Kelly, Emma Waterton, and Steve Watson, 1–11. *Critical Studies in Heritage, Emotion and Affect*. London; New York: Routledge, Taylor & Francis Group.

Vinitsky, Ilja. 2017. "Madness in Western Literature and the Arts." In *The Routledge History of Madness and Mental Health*, edited by Greg Eghigian, 153–71. London; New York: Routledge, Taylor & Francis Group.

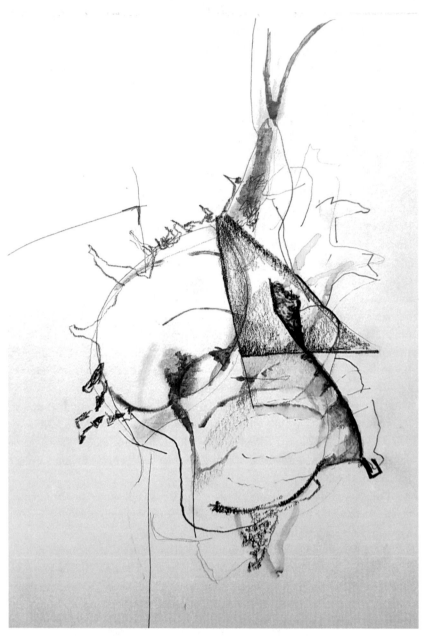

FIGURE 0.1   Marta Wandt

CHAPTER 1

Artist's Statement

Marta Wandt

I grew up in Tanzania among missionaries. Before we went to Africa, my parents went away on a six months course in London. My siblings stayed with my grandmother. But I was only nine months old and was left to a family my parents knew. When I was reunited with my family, I never bonded with my mother and my entire life has been characterized by the desire for a mother.

In Africa I had a daily life full of pain, trauma, violation and abuse by people close to me, that I should have been able to trust. I missed a mother who I could trust to protect me. My African nanny became my safe haven.

We were six siblings and some of us went to the mission boarding school. All weekends and holidays we were stowed into our car and drove off on safari and excursions. But even though I was part of a large family, I was a lonely and anxious child. I loved being by myself in our garden, dreaming and fantasizing. The nature gave me respite and comfort.

My reflections and dreams created the imagery I have found as an adult. I return and perceive.

I reflect emotions and thoughts in stones, petals, pieces of bark and sea shells. It gives me strength.

To spend time with the past and subconscious creates beauty and reconciliation. The ugly becomes beautiful, creating figures and feelings in all that I observe. As in a Rorschach test. It is a peaceful reasoning.

Mom told me a few years ago that she and I used to go on the shore of Lake Victoria and collect shells and driftwood when I was a kid. I understand now why I enjoy rocks and shells so much.

Back in Sweden, my teens became difficult. At 16, I tried to kill myself. I was placed with foster parents and started taking drugs. I lived a chaotic and bohemian life. I got married, and I got pregnant.

In the summer of 1979, when I was 22, I gave birth to my fantastic daughter. It's the biggest and finest thing that ever happened to me! At 23, I fell into a depression.

It was 37 years ago and I've been sick ever since.

I have a schizoaffective disease and when I was 26, I became psychotic.

I lived alone with my daughter for 20 years.

© KONINKLIJKE BRILL BV, LEIDEN, 2025 | DOI:10.1163/9789004519848_003

Being a mother has given my life a meaning even though I have been very sick.

Today I gather things from nature. Things that have a shape or a movement that reflects something within myself. I have a stockpile of seed capsules, dried leaves, stones and other things.

I pick up an item that speaks to me and which I think expresses the feeling that I have inside at that moment. I start to draw from what I have found. It becomes a movement on the paper. Then I keep searching.

I often lose myself in the picture, and get a desperate feeling of wanting to find a structure and get a foothold.

But to quote the Swedish poet Erik Johan Stagnelius, "Chaos lives next to God" and suddenly something is born in the picture that holds it together.

I land and I lift my eyes up.

I enjoy filling the paper with colours and lines that correspond and speak to each other. Then everything becomes bright and hopeful in an organic microcosm.

My mother is 91 years old today and she and I have been reconciled for many years. I try to leave emptiness and evil behind me.

I return to when she and I collect stones on the beach, and I end these lines with a quote by Roland Barthes "Creating is decorating the mother's body."

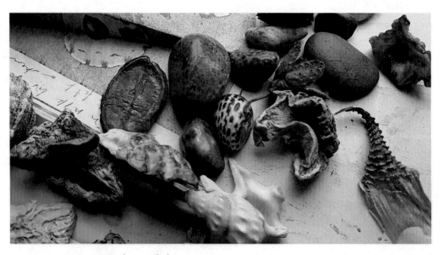

FIGURE 1.1   Marta Wandt, untitled

Unsettling the Past: Creating a Multi-Vocal Heritage of Exminster Hospital through Co-Production and Performance

Nicole Baur

Abstract

Until recently, decision-making about how heritage is understood, preserved, and therefore transmitted to future generations, has predominantly been the realm of experts and institutions. It was based on and represented through "authorised heritage discourse" (AHD) (Smith 2006) and focused around the built heritage. More recently, it has been acknowledged that heritage needs to be reconceptualised as a process and include immaterial heritage (Harvey 2001; Kirshenblatt-Gimblett 1995), as "the tangible can only be understood and interpreted through the intangible" (Munjeri 2004), with intangible heritage as the underlying framework for tangible heritage to develop value. Rather than conflicting with AHD, the new movement therefore broadens the dominant heritage discourse, as the practices embedded in AHD can be interpreted as a process of heritage making, which not only regulates the meaning of the past, but also gives meaning to group identity, historical narratives and collective and individual memories (Smith 2012, paragraph 6).

This chapter illustrates how changes in theorisation and conceptualisation of heritage can be harnessed to co-construct a multi-vocal narrative of the former Exminster Hospital near Exeter, UK. Through engaging with surviving artefacts and by embodying oral histories in workshops, people affiliated with it created new narratives that can now be passed on to future generations. The project has shown that both the hospital's material and immaterial heritage are omnipresent in the village of Exminster in buildings, street names, private archives, family genealogies as well as stories and memories. Whilst some of this heritage has been captured through AHD, complementing it with lay experiences unsettles the existing historical discourse and turns the hospital into a cultural product, offering new opportunities for interpretation and memorialisation.

© KONINKLIJKE BRILL BV, LEIDEN, 2025 | DOI:10.1163/9789004519848_004

Keywords

authorised heritage discourse – co-production – Exminster Hospital – John Charles Bucknill – mental health heritage – narrative – participatory research – Richard Eager

1   Exminster Hospital as Heritage

"The story of [Exminster] hospital is the story of the two JCBs" (EHSM02).[1] This is how my first interviewee, formerly hospital staff and by then in his nineties, introduced Exminster Hospital to me. Noticing my puzzled look, he smiled and produced two photographs. One was a black and white portrait of John Charles Bucknill, Exminster's first and unusually progressive medical super-intendent, under whom the hospital prospered in the nineteenth century. The second one – considerably younger and in colour – showed a yellow JCB digger pulling down dilapidated hospital parts. With these photographs, the interviewee had visually framed his narrative from the hospital's beginnings in 1845 through its closure in 1987 to its conversion to luxury apartments. What followed was a fascinating first-hand account of life in and around Exminster Hospital from someone who had worked there from the early 1940s to the 1980s and, as a local councillor, became involved in decisions regarding the hospital in the 1990s and 2000s. Leaving after two hours, several cups of tea, and with at least two days' worth of transcription work ahead of me, it dawned on me that although I had researched Exminster Hospital for six years, I had familiarised myself with only one narrative – the official one available in surviving records. His narrative made me even more curious about how the local community, former staff, and patients felt about the hospital. What personal experiences and memories would I uncover? What did the hospital mean to them? My aim was not to produce a "counter-story" – although some accounts I heard diverge greatly from official records – but to learn about the hospital and its material and immaterial legacy from people who were directly affected by it, but whose voices could – at best – be discovered between the lines of official documents.

For decades, heritage – including mental health heritage – has been selected according to the "authorised heritage discourse" (Smith 2006), thus prioritis-ing material remnants of the past. When Exminster Hospital closed, the prem-ises lay vacant, suffering severe decay before being rescued in the early 2000s. Its material heritage remains easily recognisable. Its immaterial heritage

---

1   For confidentiality reasons, project participants are referred to by the codes allocated to
     them.

is much more difficult to grasp, as this is constructed based on the various meanings and emotions people directly affected by it attached to it. Exploring these meanings has been facilitated by a growing interest in immaterial heritage, such as "oral expressions" and "social practices" (UNESCO 2003), which emerged from the 1980s' cultural turn (Warren-Findley 2013). This so-called "democratisation" of heritage has therefore resulted in opportunities to create a multi-vocal representation of the past – both in analogue and digital forms – and a welcome diversion from reducing history to a single narrative (Massey 1995). Critics, however, argue that this discourse is yet underexplored (Smith 2013). Indeed – with some notable exceptions (Goffman 1973; Jones 1972; Ryan and Thomas 1980) – asylum historiographies have tended to focus on buildings, hierarchies, and legislation. Advocates of this new movement therefore call for "a new approach to cultural heritage, one that is participatory, bottom-up and fundamentally grounded in local concerns and interests" (Schofield 2014, 2). More recent calls go further, demanding the re-conceptualisation of heritage as a process (Duncan 1995; Kirshenblatt-Gimblett 1998; Heumann 2006; Smith 2006; Andermann and Arnold de Simine 2012), thereby allowing for the co-existence of multiple, parallel, contradictory, or even contested narratives (Smith 2006) and enabling much-needed critique with regards to privileging some accounts over others. This is not an easy task for anyone, lest academic researchers engaging in participatory research who have to balance aims of community participation and co-production against the expectations of academic peer review processes integral to grant applications and publishing outcomes. Consequently, even projects striving for co-creation are influenced by the researcher with regards to what heritage is to be preserved, how it is preserved, and who will have access to it.

This chapter seeks to contribute to this discourse with a participatory approach to the heritage of Exminster Hospital. The project the chapter is based on gave a voice to those people whose ambivalent experiences of Exminster Hospital have been marginalised in the existing official discourse. By focusing on immaterial heritage, it uncovered meanings, emotions, and narratives that stayed in participants' minds for decades, but will disappear with these people's passing, if not captured. It illustrated that the hospital was subject to multiple – sometimes conflicting, but predominantly complementary – narratives of daily hospital life, not just those officially documented and transferred to archives in order to be passed on to future generations. Following a description of the project underpinning this chapter, including a methodological statement, the chapter focuses on three heritage narratives describing life within the hospital and its connections with the local community.

2   "Remembering the Mental Hospital" – a Participatory Approach to
         Exminster Hospital's Heritage

The history of former "lunatic asylums", such as Exminster Hospital, has been
explored by social historians, historians of psychiatry and those interested in
the architecture of these buildings – frequently informed by and in dialogue
with the works of Erving Goffman (1973) and Michel Foucault (1979) and predominantly guided by surviving official records. "Remembering the Mental
Hospital" took a different, but complementary, approach inspired by the recognition that the hospital's surviving physical landmarks, which are memorials to
the current generation affiliated with the hospital, will soon lose this meaning
unless they are accompanied by people's narratives. The project therefore set
out to combine the hospital's material and immaterial heritage and to generate
intergenerational dialogue by bringing together former staff, patients, members from the local community of all ages. Participatory in nature, the project's
focus was on co-production. Exminster Hospital's physical landmarks were
used both as settings to evoke memories and narratives, and as places where
new material and immaterial heritage was created. Accessibility to project
outcomes was facilitated through presentations at local history societies, interactive exhibitions, and a website. The latter allows people across the world to
engage with heritage narratives of the hospital without being physically present at the hospital premises or the local archives – albeit with certain legal
constraints and copyright regulations.

3   Sources and Methods: Co-Constructing Narratives of Exminster
         Hospital's Heritage

Asylum historiographers have privileged official records owing to other sources
being less easily available. With the closure of large mental hospitals, memories
and personal experiences of people affiliated with them have become valuable sources of immaterial heritage beyond these accounts. Oral histories are
increasingly used as a means to oppose the elite "voices of the past" (Thompson 1978), as they provide a perspective "from below" and give insights into a
world that was produced and consumed in complex and multiple ways (e.g.
Smith and Jackson 1999; Summerfield 2004). They are, however, highly problematic strands of data for three reasons. Firstly, oral history is not simply the
recollection of the storyteller, but the "shared authority" of both interviewer
and interviewee, who jointly create the testimony (Frisch 1990). Thus, they
are partial, subjective, reflexive, ambiguous, sometimes contradictory and

often tensioned (Bender 2004). Secondly, oral histories often include memories, which are fluid and influenced by people's life experiences. Thus, as with other forms of history, they do not always represent past events accurately and should not be used as the sole gateway to the past. Finally, oral histories do not necessarily provide a voice for people with difficulties articulating themselves verbally.

"Remembering the Mental Hospital" addressed these caveats by combining oral histories, written lay narratives, photovoice (Baur 2017), photo-reminiscence, soundwalks (Schafer 1977) and arts activities in order to paint a more nuanced picture of Exminster Hospital's heritage and engage new generations with it. Combining methods – particularly oral histories and photovoice with creative activities, such as writing or arts workshops, is not only becoming more frequent in qualitative social research, but moving away from traditional research – and dissemination – methods is crucial in participatory research due to the unfamiliarity of participants with academic research practices. This development has been facilitated by recent advances in technology, including mobile phones with sound recording options and high-quality cameras.

The above outlined combination of data collection was deemed particularly suitable for a project applying a participatory approach, as it allowed for a multi-sensory experience of the hospital. Moreover, it enabled people less able to articulate themselves verbally to participate. As people engaged with the physical heritage of Exminster Hospital, they recounted numerous individual stories that formed the narrative of the hospital, which, complemented – and sometimes contradicted – the official narrative. Narrative, in this project, was both, a method of capturing data and a type of project output. Rather than being limited to its usual restrictive temporal sense, spatial components formed an integral part of the narrative, thereby bestowing it with the power to become an active element in the social production of space and place. This way, the work also contributes to cross-disciplinary research in oral history and geography, an area largely neglected in existing academic publications. "Narrative interviewing" allowed participants to tell their own stories after being prompted by an overarching question/theme or a visual artefact. Interviewing took place in participants' homes, but also as walking interviews and sound walks on the hospital's premises. Participants who were too frail to join walks, but wanted to participate in group activities, were invited to arts workshops and photovoice sessions (Baur 2017). Here, conversations were also recorded and, as all soundbites, transcribed verbatim, i.e. including all verbal and non-verbal cues. Interview transcripts were reviewed with the participants in follow-up sessions to ensure they accurately reflected the stories and to address gaps, silences, or apparent contradictions. This way, participants became active collaborators in creating the narratives. Audio-recordings and transcripts have been passed on to a local archive to be made publicly accessible in line with UK data protection legislation. In total, 32 participants were interviewed. Contents of the interviews served as basis for a public exhibition, creative arts and drama workshops conducted at the hospital premises as well as a local primary school. Snippets and short quotes from oral histories were also used to inspire the photo-reminiscence sessions and soundwalks in order to create a multi-sensory experience. In addition to following a route guided by sound bites from oral histories, participants were also encouraged to record their own sounds and thoughts along the way. The experience gained from such soundwalks was later discussed in workshops, which encouraged participants to share their experience and simultaneously acted as a key to the past, triggering memories which turned into narratives and stories. Data analysis was carried out using NVIVO (Version 11), as this was deemed the best method to do justice to such diverse types of data.

Findings reveal that the (hi)story of Exminster Hospital is by no means as clear-cut as the official historiography of such institutions suggests. The former asylum was a place of dichotomies, had different meanings for different people, and aroused different feelings and emotions. In co-producing narratives with people whose histories contributed to making up Exminster Hospital's heritage, "Remembering the Mental Hospital" increases the relevance of this heritage to younger generations, helping them to connect with the people and places Exminster Village commemorates and preserves in street names and other material objects. In the following sections some of these meanings and emotions will be explored and discussed based on three heritage narratives: Exminster Hospital as a treatment centre, Exminster Hospital and stigma, and the Exminster community.

4   Heritage Narrative 1: Exminster Hospital as a Treatment Centre

Exminster Hospital opened in August 1845 and was amongst the first institutions dedicated to pauper patients before the 1845 Lunacy Act rendered hospitals for pauper patients mandatory. Intended as "a place where curative treatment is applied [...] not a place of confinement or punishment" (Devon Minute Book 1844), its design and layout mirrored the latest therapeutic knowledge (Baur 2019). Its first Medical Superintendent, the above-mentioned John Charles Bucknill, turned Exminster Hospital into one of the UK's most progressive county asylums of the time, which earned him an international reputation beyond Europe. His material legacy are the numerous articles in international journals, and pamphlets housed at the local archive. Bucknill also initiated medical research, which continued at Exminster throughout its life-course. From trialling sedatives in the nineteenth century, the hospital moved towards the more invasive shock treatments (including Cardiazol, Insulin and Electric Shock Treatments) when the 1930s Mental Treatment Act (Jones 1960) encouraged such research. One such therapy still remembered by project participants was malaria treatment for psychosis: "The mosquito was used on people and Exminster was a centre. The train [came] in [from London] and staff was sent to pick up the bottles with the mosquitoes, which stung through the muslin" (EHSM12). Surviving archival documents attest to the delivery by train – as well as to the frantic search for a box of mosquitoes which had gone astray on the transport.[2] Whether these mosquitoes were successfully retrieved, remains a mystery. Being at the forefront of contemporary medical research, however, came with its own downsides, as patients regularly doubled up as "human guinea pigs". Exminster patients undergoing malaria therapy, for instance, unwittingly supported a League of Nations' trial to compare the efficacy of various anti-malarial agents, which advanced the hospital's reputation at the time (James 1933).

Starting in the 1930s, malaria therapy was replaced by shock therapies (Baur 2013). Short trials with Cardiazol shock therapy were succeeded by Insulin and Electric shock treatments in the late 1930s and early 1940s. These are still vividly remembered by project participants, their accounts attesting to their ambivalence towards them. Whilst their accounts might seem contradictory in places, they give us a more nuanced picture of these therapies and their impact on patients and staff than existing historiographies based on surviving administrative records. They also reveal that understanding how these therapies worked was rudimentary at the best – even amongst contemporary doctors:

> it did work in some cases, but I don't think they knew what they were doing. [...] Electrical treatment was in vogue for many years. I regarded the early forms of that as barbaric. But later-on it became recognised – and I am told it benefited [some people] for a time (EHSM02).

Exminster introduced Insulin Coma Therapy (ICT) in 1937. One former staff reflects:

> Insulin therapy, these patients were very compliant, sort of dulled down. What did they do? They [gave] them an injection and they were all very overweight, bloated people, because [of] the diet they were given and

---

2   Uncatalogued correspondence, Devon Record Office, Exeter.

the lack of exercise – and they thought it would change the way their brains worked, I suppose. So, they had this injection and then they'd be monitored and they'd be in an almost deep coma and then they'd put a nasal-gastric tube in and lots of glucose and they used to wake up very rapidly. It was quite horrible, really. Yes, it was horrible. And they were pretty zombie-like people (EHSF21).

Electro-Convulsive Therapy (ECT) joined ICT, and staff began to recognise adverse effects associated with it:

Why have they got loss of memory? It was because they had had so much ECT. It absolutely fried their brains. It was a frightful thing. In the very beginning, the spasm was so violent, they would fracture their spines. And then they gave them a muscle-relaxant. I've watched that as a student and that was pretty terrifying because the person – it relaxed you, so it relaxed your intercostal muscle, so you didn't breathe. So, you couldn't let that go on for very long before you whacked on the thing – bzzzz, you know, and a massive spasm, I can sort of see it now. The whole body, absolutely everything went into a massive spasm and relaxed and then oxygen quickly and bring them out of it, you know. It was very primitive, it really was (EHSF21).

Accidents – and sometimes also deaths – did occur in Exminster as a result of shock treatments and entered the official records. The Medical Superintendent downplayed the incidents, as in the case of one patient who suffered broken bones from ECT treatment, but was "now up and about in a plaster jacket [and] quite comfortable".[3] In fact, a number of Medical Superintendents from the 1920s to the 1940s were delighted with the perceived progress in apparent cures that led to many discharges: "with the more enlightened treatment of patients, many were the new departures in the years between the wars" (Allan 1945).

Many project participants, in contrast, revealed that the (often failing) treatments impacted negatively on them, a fact usually omitted from asylum historiographies. One former nurse, for instance, recalls accompanying patients to ECT:

You [took] them to the room and they used to lay them down and give them an injection, put this thing in their mouth, and then they put a

---

3   Medical Superintendent's Monthly Reports, Devon Record Office, March & April 1944.

blanket over them and stand clear and put a thing on their heads and shock them. When they came 'round we used to give them a cup of tea … that wasn't very nice. The doctors were … it was just clinical (EHSM05).

Others regretted not having the courage to speak up for the patients:

Once it was over he was pushed into the recovery room and I sat with him and when he opened his eyes, his pupils were huge and he was like a rabbit in the headlights. I was frightened – not of him, but I was frightened of what had been done to him. I wish I had spoken up for him, been his advocate, not just an observer. And if this is how they did it in the [19]80s, what the hell was it like in the [19]50s? (EHSF09).

There were, however, also success stories:

I can remember a patient who was acutely depressed. She was thirty, thirty-five, something like that, and wouldn't eat, wouldn't do anything, just sit there and mope. She wouldn't speak, just gazed into your eyes. We got a drip in 'cause she was getting dehydrated, she'd rip it out. Got a tube in, she'd pull it out. So, we wondered what else we could do? She'd come to the stage that if she'd been left a few more days, she'd have died of dehydration. So, we gave her ECT. We gave her about three shots on Tuesday, Friday and the following Tuesday, and she started responding. Within a short while she was eating and much better, couldn't believe what she had been through" (EHSF07). Other staff acknowledge that ECT benefited some people: "[W]e had ECT, which again is something that sounds barbaric. But I've also seen some people when they started to be very concerned about giving ECT, suffered greatly mentally for the lack of any other treatment that actually worked for them. So, I think it has to be seen in the wider scope rather than – and things have obviously progressed (EHSF14).

The state-of-the-art treatment could come at a cost – both emotionally for staff and sometimes life-changing for patients. Furthermore, whilst the willingness (and also financial means) was there to trial novel invasive treatments, this often came at the expense of less invasive treatments, such as Occupational Therapy (OT), which was introduced in Exminster in the 1930s by Dr Richard Eager. Similar to Bucknill, he gained international reputation, hosting delegates from as far as the USA to familiarise themselves with this novel form of treatment. World War II brought an abrupt end to OT and its re-introduction after the War was slow in the then cash-strapped and overcrowded hospital. Project participants reminisced how the few OTs pulled together with other staff and the local community to provide such activities for the patients:

> in the beginning we got people gardening. There was a very nice garden there. I begged the League of Friends for some money for chickens. So, we had some hens and we sold – well, the idea was that we would sell our eggs. It didn't work because people pinched them all the time, but still, the idea was alright. So, suddenly there was some purposeful activity, which is what OT is all about. So, then what else would I do? I had other ideas. I wanted a goat and I was offered a goat and I was quite excited about my goat. But one of the psychiatrists had this concern about these deprived men and my little goat and what might happen to it – so, I wasn't allowed to have my goat. It was quite sad, but probably would have been quite difficult to deal with anyway (EHSF21).

Whilst many published accounts have dealt with the topic of treatments in mental hospitals, the focus has often been on the lack of treatment, the use of treatment for doctors to further their own careers, or on treatment as a means to "normalise" people. Narratives gained from this project complement these publications by adding the perspective of the people who were actually involved in administering the treatments and caring for the patients who had received them. In doing so, they add a different perspective of daily life within mental hospitals. Fun and laughter absolutely existed, as did strong ties between staff and patients and amongst staff members themselves. Exminster Hospital was originally designed to be a place of healing for people suffering from mental distress, and findings show that staff put great effort into living up to these standards. It also faced prejudice and stigma, but, as will be shown below, such sentiments were generally restricted to people unaffiliated with the hospital. "Remembering the Mental Hospital" – through giving agency to people historically excluded from asylum historiographies – paints a complementary picture, thereby advancing our collective understanding of mental health care heritage.

5   Heritage Narrative 2: Exminster Hospital and Stigma

One might assume that a place that prides itself of offering state-of-the-art treatment would be held in high regard by patients. Instead, like many psychiatric institutions, Exminster Hospital suffered from the stigma attached to mental distress and its places of treatment. During the hospital's existence, mental health and distress was rarely openly discussed and misunderstanding, prejudice, confusion and fear frequently resulted in discrimination of patients and their relatives. Many Exminster patients were rarely visited and some never returned to their families and communities for fear of being ostracised. Those who did often found it difficult to re-integrate into their communities – both socially and in the workplace. Published literature often attributes stigma to the certification process which, up to the 1930 Mental Treatment Act, was the only route into a mental hospital. The sources used for this chapter, however, tell a slightly different story, confirming that many patients and their relatives alike felt uneasy about the hospital, but simultaneously providing novel insights about the reasons for this uneasiness. These can be subdivided into fears of the place itself and the treatment provided therein, its residents and staff, but also the community and its often discriminatory reactions towards patients and relatives. The interconnectedness of these types of fear makes disentangling them extremely difficult.

In many cases Exminster's "good reputation", which survived into the post-World War II world defying overcrowding and underfunding, and the overwhelming trust in the medical staff there compensated for the stigma of having been admitted:

> It was a great shock to me when I received your notice that my daughter has been admitted to your hospital. The more so as I had not been consulted. At first, I felt angry and inclined to take her away at once, but on second thoughts I felt a gentleman of Dr [Name] standing would not do anything detrimental to the patients' best interests. If you start her on the high road to recovery it will more than compensate for the 'stigma' or supposed stigma.[4]

Indeed, close analyses of correspondence between patients' relatives and Exminster Hospital show that many relatives, who up to the 1960s had to consent to patients' treatment, explicitly asked for the treatments described above to be applied to the patients, desperately hoping for a cure.

Although the above quote mentions "stigma", it is unclear from the correspondence, whether this is attached to Exminster Hospital as a place or whether it arises from suffering from mental distress and seeking treatment.

---

4   Uncatalogued correspondence by WP, 21/07/1941, Devon Record Office.

More explicit in this respect is the following quote, illustrating that even with their best efforts, staff have been unable to elucidate reasons for visitors refusing to come to Exminster:

> I have been unable to persuade any of the members of the family to visit Mr [*Name*] here – they say they would visit him in Redhills or the City Hospital, but not in Exminster [Hospital], and none of them was intelligent enough to voice their fears about the place (EHSF13).

Yet, even here it cannot be said for sure, whether the uneasiness was caused by the place or the people treated there. Fears of patients existed within the community as well as amongst fellow patients. As the following quote reveals, this often resulted from lack of knowledge about mental distress and how to deal with people affected by it:

> you would have somebody in and nobody would visit or anything and you'd ring a next of kin and say "look, the person is very, very ill" – [...] that was very tragic, to think that somebody ended their life with none of their relatives around them. That was horrible" (EHSF19). Reflecting on the above statement, another participant sought to explain the behaviour: "I am wondering if it was the stigma or because they were confused, they didn't know how to talk to them. They were embarrassed, you know [...] You'd have relatives and they'd be quite aggressive towards the staff and, if you got underneath that, it's embarrassment. And "why my father, why my mother" and all this (EHSF08).

The hospital and its inhabitants evoked feelings of uneasiness amongst the local community and hospital staff alike. One lady recalls riding her bicycle as a young girl:

> when we came up to Exminster Hospital, we always pedalled a bit faster to go past because there were always these people standing around, at the gates, and some of them were mental patients. They were drooling. I know they couldn't help it, but – [... it was] just a bit scary (EHSF16).

A former employee adds:

> patients used to wander the corridor – there was one guy who used to brush the corridors every day. It was all repetitive stuff, but he used to brush the corridors every day and you tended – *I* tended – in my first

few weeks to walk around, looking over my shoulder all the time until I started to feel comfortable (EHSF18).

Although we do not know whether these patients' appearances and habits were part of their distress or consequences of the hospital treatment, some of the treatments described above had visible impacts, exposing patients physically as such to others whilst simultaneously leaving them to cope with their changed selves. Looking back, staff agree that their fear of patients usually disappeared very quickly under the right guidance and training and many have very fond memories of patients. Similarly, as the hospital opened its doors in the 1950s, many patients became valued members of the Exminster Village community, frequenting the local pub and doing odd jobs for the villagers.

In addition, more in-depth conversations about fear and stigma revealed that much of it was socially founded. As many small villages in rural Devon, Exminster is a close-knit community where everybody knew everybody. Furthermore, many villagers worked at the hospital:

> It must have been embarrassing to my uncle that he was in there, I was working there, and another of his nieces – no, two nieces – were working there. One was a ward sister" (EHSM27). Another participant recalled: "You know, with the stigma the families never used to come up, a lot of them they didn't. I looked after one lady on one of the wards, which she was put in because she was pregnant and not married. And it was really sad because she had family in the Village [Exminster]. And her niece used to work at the Hospital. Never came to see her (EHSM27).

The above narration illustrates that in addition to the public stigma, i.e. the reaction of outsiders towards people suffering from mental distress, many patients also felt embarrassed about their distress and the "trouble" they were causing to their families. This situation may be better understood in the context of the next quote, which describes how being treated at Exminster impacted on the lives of the patients and their families long after their discharge:

> my uncle shouldn't have been in there. I think he was saner than me [*laughs*], but because he couldn't get a job – and the problem was, when they got in there, there was a big stigma and nobody wanted them out. That was the real end of it (EHSM27).

Correspondence reveals that some families became upset at the prospect of having their relative return back home to them. One husband, for example, requested for his wife to be transferred to another hospital before her death, anticipating stigma and fearing for his children's future:

> Would it be possible for her to be transferred to another hospital for to have special treatment for what she is suffering from and also for her children's sake if anything should happen to her, so that it can't be said that she passed away in a mental hospital.[5]

The husband's anxiety shows that the stigma was not only attached to the person suffering from mental ill-health, but could be extended to include their entire family. In a rural county like Devon with predominantly small villages and close-knit communities, stereotypes and misconceptions attached to mental distress and people seeking mental health care could therefore severely hamper relatives' future quality of life.

6   Heritage Narrative 3: "The Hospital Was the Village and the Village Was the Hospital" – the Exminster Community

With a few notable exceptions (Gittens 1998), historiographies describe psychiatric hospitals as oppressive places dominated by hierarchies, strict social control and tightly regulated timetables (e.g. Foucault 1979; Goffman 1973; Rothman 2001). Whilst this is in part true for Exminster, our project participants who used to work at the hospital allowed us to get more in-depth knowledge of the daily working life within the hospital and its connections to Exminster Village.

Participants describe Exminster Hospital as "a community by itself" (EHSF01), a place where "everybody knew everybody [...] like a family" (EHSF17). This made it a safe and comfortable place, as people could rely on each other. Such comforts were added to by the fact that "the pay was good, the social life was brilliant" (EHSF24). It also provided a certain amount of freedom. Young female nurses who would never have entered a pub on their own, for example, could go to the hospital's social club. These feelings were often conveyed in comparison to the NHS since the 1990s, as many staff who transferred to community care after the closure of the hospital missed exactly this support. This community spirit is still apparent when many former staff meet for an annual Christmas dinner. It also impacted on patients: "You do

---

5   Uncatalogued correspondence by JS, 08/09/1948, Devon Record Office.

get relationships with people because you'd know people for such a long time. And also, the people that would become ill from the Village, you'd know their family" (EHSF02). Some participants feel that this close-knittedness had an element of surveillance. Nobody would have been able to drink underage in the social club, for example, because everyone knew who they were and how old they were. Furthermore, "you had to be very careful who you made friends with or who you were bitchy about because there were lots of families" (EHSF21). But as one former nurse sums it up: "but then that was the Village. Yes, it was great fun" (EHSFR06).

Staff agree that working at Exminster Hospital was demanding and also challenging at times. Simultaneously, it was a place of great humour and fun involving both patients and staff:

> I had a phone call – Cornwall Police, very stern voice. He said "does your hospital have a tug used for conveying food around the Hospital?" – "Yes" – he said "did you know that it's passing Lympstone Barracks at the moment? It's going at five miles per hour. We've apprehended the driver and he says he wanted to go and have a swim (EHSM02).

Neither the tug nor the patient driving it had been missed at all. Another staff recounted that training as a doctor on Hallett Clinic was particularly popular during the summer months:

> they used [*Hallett Clinic*] as a training ward for doctors. You'd get all sorts, all different nationalities. And a lot of them were coming in the summer because of the cricket team – you could watch the cricket from out of the window from the ward and then the doctors used to come in watching the cricket. You'd often find them missing and they'd be up there watching it (EHSF02).

The fun also brought distraction to the patients:

> There was a staff nurse full of life. It was a quiet time and she was messing around. So, I thought "I'll get you". We made a bodice of newspaper wrapped with Sellotape around her and a skirt and got this disposable bedpan with a pyjama cord to make a hat and made spots on it and she went into the lounge. There was this elderly lady who was so miserable, she really didn't crack her face at all. She was standing up on her Zimmer frame, looked at her, and rocked with laughter, absolutely rocked. And, she never forgot that. She was a different woman after that. She smiled, there

was something that struck a chord with her. And if we [had] got into trouble it was worth it because that made such a difference to that lady and also her care because we were able to communicate with her (EHSF14).

The Exminster community also included children of staff and villagers. Their experiences and memories are of particular interest, as they illustrate that, on the one hand, they were free to roam the vast grounds of the hospital, which was greatly enjoyed. On the other hand, however, they were confronted with hospital life from a very early age, as what was going on within the hospital was often taken home by their parents and discussed around the dinner table.

Many children recall going up to the hospital almost daily to visit their parents who were working there (EHSF22). Others remember walking across the hospital fields on their daily walk to the village school (EHSM05) and using the hospital premises for their afternoon activities:

> it was a mine of activity around there with all the different buildings. And we used to play in the yard, the farm yard, when the cattle had gone and all the fencing was taken down to give us more wiggle area. Ya, cowboys and Indians around the farm buildings. And as we grew up, we got interested in the football and cricket, and they are probably one of the best sets of playing fields in the county. We often went down there and played at night quite late, straight from school (EHSM05).

Whilst this participant did not seem to have any concerns regarding the hospital or its residents, other quotes rebalance this testimony by acknowledging that there were limits to the freedom children had on the premises:

> there were some wards that we weren't allowed to go into, but I do remember going in from time to time to see my mum and, you know, they had the fantastic farm there which we used to go to see the pigs and things like that. We'd play cricket on the cricket field – it was somewhere where we just, you know, we had various places where we cycled, and the hospital was one of those places. I don't think we ever felt any fear or intimidation (EHSF30).

From this particular quote, we cannot elucidate what the ban from certain wards was based on and whether it was to protect the children or whether it might simply have been locked wards accessible to authorised medical staff only. It is clear, however, that there was no general ban between patients and the children, as patients used to work on the farm and the stables, so children would have met them when they visited the pigs or played cricket. As the following quote suggests, people unaffiliated with the hospital might have been frightened of the patients, but having relatives working at the hospital dispersed the fears:

> I wasn't frightened, which I think some people were. Maybe that's the people that relatives there that were more frightened of the whole thing. Because it was where [my relatives] worked and if it was alright for them, then it was alright for me as a child. My perception of it wasn't frightening (EHSF09).

Being so involved with the hospital *did* mean, however, that, even at home, children could not escape hospital life:

> My mother, my father and my sister and my step-father all worked at Exminster Hospital. And I remember sitting around the dinner table, that would be the only topic of conversation – the Hospital. And I used to say, even as a small child, "can we just talk about something else, please, instead of Exminster bloody Hospital? (EHSF30).

Despite the community spirit, hierarchies and regulations existed at Exminster. These included segregation according to professional rank: "the Sisters used to go for breakfast in the Nurses' Home and sit on one table, the Staff Nurses on the other, the SEN on another. They wouldn't mix" (EHSF25). Others remember that Sisters and Matrons would not even look at the lower-ranked nurses when talking to them. Such hierarchical systems could be intimidating, particularly for younger nurses, and were not always appreciated:

> when the Matron came through, you stood to attention. It was awful. Didn't matter what you were doing with a patient, you had to stop and look at the Matron and say "Good Morning" or "Good Afternoon". It was – to me, that was very shocking because to me, if you are looking after people, the people you are looking after come first (EHSF08).

The nurses developed their own strategies to deal with these situations. One recalled that they were strictly forbidden to have their tea break on the wards. It was often impossible to leave the wards, however, because of staff shortages and patient overcrowding. Coating the steps to the ward with sugar meant they would hear the Matron arrive and had enough time to hide their cups of tea and biscuits.

Several participants have also reported a blurring of hierarchies and segregation between staff and patients. This took place in the recreational spaces such as the Ballroom and the sports facilities, as has been discussed elsewhere (Baur 2017). Events held in these spaces were also frequently attended by villagers. Another place where staff and patients mixed was the "Stowey Arms", the village pub that was frequented by both groups alike.

When the hospital closed in 1987, staff got redeployed to the many small community treatment centres around the county of Devon. One felt that with the closure of the hospital much of the community disappeared as well:

> As a villager and Nurse living in Exminster I observed and recorded the physical change to the hospital as parts of it were demolished to make way for new houses, roads and layouts and how other parts were saved and re-developed. I was aware too of the loosening association the village had with the former hospital as the dispersal of staff and patients gathered apace and increasingly all that remained was the shell of the former hospital and as the re-development gathered momentum soon the physical structure lost some of its predominance over the landscape (EHSM12).

But as was stated above, this feeling is not shared by everyone as some of this community continues to exist in the annual meetings.

7   Conclusion

Unlike many of its contemporaries, key buildings and garden features of Exminster Hospital survived because they could be repurposed. Together with these material landmarks, official records survived, based on which the heritage of the hospital can be reconstructed. They narrate, however, only one story. By applying a participatory approach and combining sources such as correspondence, oral histories, photovoice, photo-reminiscence, soundwalks and arts activities, all of which have so far received insufficient attention, this chapter has shown that there are multiple narratives which all contribute to creating a more nuanced heritage of the hospital.

Exminster Hospital's physical heritage has been preserved across the village in buildings and street names. Contrary to commemorative monuments, street names have not only symbolic functions, but also practical ones as geographical markers for spatial orientation. In this latter function, they encourage daily engagement with history. Street names commemorating Exminster Hospital's heritage include a variety of people and features affiliated with the hospital, not least because much of the naming was achieved on the incentive of the local population: "When it came to the land being sold and the roads being named, I took major part in naming roads on the estate after people who had made their name in the Hospital. So, Pridham's Way is after a Matron, and after my old boss Douglas Miller, Miller Way is named after him. So, those names are significant" (EHSM08). Ivy Pridham started at Exminster as a student nurse in the 1920s and worked her way up to Matron. She is remembered by many project participants for ruling of the wards with an iron fist. Interestingly, she is the only female staff who had a street named after her. Several street names refer to doctors, amongst them Medical Superintendent Bucknill (Bucknill Close, Brownlees, Eager Close, Penny Close) and the famous architect of the hospital, Charles Fowler (Fowler Close). Holley Close is named after the once hospital-owned Holley Cottages, which were demolished in order to make room for the new development after the closure of the hospital. Other names commemorate the still-existing lime trees lining "the Drive", i.e. the approach to Exminster Hospital, giving it a stately appearance (Lime Grove, Lime Cottages) and the Reddaway family whose member Tom Reddaway was Clerk of Works at Exminster Hospital. Using this material heritage as a setting for events and activities has revealed that it abounds with elements that evoke memories and stories, which constitute important parts of its immaterial heritage. Information gathered throughout the project illustrated that the hospital's immaterial heritage is, in fact, even stronger than its material one, and has, over the past century, become an important feature of village life and culture. So much, that even more than three decades after the hospital's closure, the phrase "to go up the 'sylum" is still used amongst residents of Exminster village when talking about walking up the hill where the now luxury estate is located. Furthermore, existing remembrance includes urban legend, for example, the premises being haunted by ghosts as well as a booklet written by community members which celebrates buildings as well as former staff and patients (Rawlinson n.d.). However, the memories discussed in our project and presented in this chapter are individual and there have only been limited efforts to capture and turn them into memorials. Hence, these immaterial elements will die with their owners and, over time, weaken Exminster Hospital's material heritage, as future generations will lose the connection created through these narratives. The project underpinning this chapter therefore aimed to combine material and immaterial heritage in order to create narratives that can be passed on to future generations. This combination illustrates that progress in mental health care was by no means linear over the past century and that what was perceived to be "progressive" by some could trigger anxiety in others – and might even have prevented some people from seeking help. Staff accounts discussed in this chapter attest to the importance of entering into dialogue and creating rapport with patients, as this – together with active participation in their treatment process – are important elements of achieving well-being.

As all narratives, the ones presented in this chapter have to be understood as conflating past events influenced by the narrators' background and experiences with individual choices. As such, they prioritise some people or events over others – many of which have not been taken into account by the dominant asylum narratives. Gaps in these dominant narratives have opened the door for alternative ones, which at first glance, might undermine the authority of the dominant narratives, but, at closer look, rather complement these by adding perspectives and allowing people to create their own understanding of the past. Combining the narratives from "Remembering the Mental Hospital" with the dominant asylum historiographies therefore paints a picture that more truly represents the heritage of mental health care and has the capacity to carry it on to a broader community without a direct link to Exminster Hospital.

At a cursory glance, Exminster Hospital does not differ so much from existing historiographies of other former psychiatric hospitals. Similar to them, it was intended to be a therapeutic place, but any treatment offered was not only dependent the state of therapeutic knowledge, but also influenced by cash, capacity, and the initiative of the medical superintendent in charge. It was also a highly stigmatised, and stigmatizing, place and work was guided by hierarchies and regulations. Rather than counteracting these official narratives, participants' accounts add to them important elements omitted so far. These include, for instance, the impact of available treatments on staff and patients and reasons for avoiding the hospital. They also show the community spirit and humour amongst staff and between staff and patients. Fostering relationships – some of which lasted beyond hospitalisation – could be as therapeutic as medical treatment. What feelings and emotions were triggered throughout the project – and therefore what narratives emerged from our engagement with participants – seemed to depend on the environment participants were in (both social and physical), the materials and objects used during the sessions, participants' previous positions and the spaces they inhabited within the hospital, as well as their prior knowledge of the hospital. This chapter therefore calls for a more careful selection of sources earmarked for retention – and for the inclusion of narratives and experiences of people who have largely been disenfranchised in existing accounts – as they contribute considerably to our understanding of the heritage of psychiatric institutions.

References

Allan, S. 1945. *Devon Mental Hospital 1845–1945. The History of the Hospital*. N.p.

Andermann, Jens, and Silke Arnold-de Simine. 2012. "Introduction: Memory, Community and the New Museum." *Theory, Culture & Society* 29 (1): 3–13. https://doi .org/10.1177/0263276411423041.

Baur, Nicole. 2013. "Family influence and psychiatric care: Physical treatments in Devon mental hospitals, c. 1920 to the 1970s." *Endeavour* 37 (3): 172–83. https://doi .org/.org/ https://doi.org/10.1016/j.endeavour (accessed June 06, 2013).

Baur, Nicole. 2017. "Exminster Hospital explored through photovoice and digital storytelling." *Sozialraum.de*. https://www.sozialraum.de/exminster-hospital-explored -through-photovoice-and-digital-storytelling-a-participatory-approach.php (accessed June 11, 2020).

Baur, Nicole. 2019. "'This Weather Always Gets Me Down': A Psychosocial Perspective on Mental Illness." *Health* 23 (2): 180–96. https://doi.org/.org/10.1177/1363459318804602.

Bender, Barbara. 2004. "The Branscombe Project: Where History Meets Memory." Paper presented at "Talking Landscapes: On Geography and the Practice of Oral History", University of Exeter, UK, July 08, 2004.

Devon Minute Book, 1844, uncatalogued booklet, Devon Record Office, Exeter.

Duncan, Carol. 2005. *Civilizing Rituals*. London: Routledge.

Foucault, Michel. 1967. *Madness and Civilization: A History of Insanity in the Age of Reason*. London: Tavistock.

Frisch, Michael. 1990. *A Shared Authority: Essays on the Craft and Meaning of Oral and Public History*. SUNY Series in Oral and Public History. State University of New York Press.

Gittens, Diane. 1998. *Madness in its place: narratives of Severalls Hospital 1913–1997*. London: Routledge.

Goffman, Erving. 1961. *Asylums: Essays on the Social Situations of Mental Patients and Other Inmates.*Oxford, England: Doubleday (Anchor).

Harvey, David C. 2001. "Heritage Pasts and Heritage Presents: Temporality, Meaning and the Scope of Heritage Studies." *International Journal of Heritage Studies* 7 (4): 319–38. https://doi.org/10.1080/13581650120105534.

Heumann Gurian, Elaine. 2006. *Civilizing the Museum*. London: Routledge. https://doi .org/10.4324/9780203003565.

James, S. 1933. "Antimalarial Chemotherapeutic Tests at the Devon Mental Hospital." *Journal of Tropical Medicine & Hygiene* 36: 289–91.

Jones, Kathleen. 1972. "A History of the Mental Health Services." London: Routledge & Kegan Paul.

Jones, Kathleen. 2013. 1960. *Mental Health and Social Policy, 1845–1959*. London: Routledge. https://doi.org/10.4324/9781315008301.

Kirshenblatt-Gimblett, Barbara. 1995. "Theorizing Heritage." *Ethnomusicology* 39 (3): 367–80. https://doi.org/10.2307/924627.

Kirshenblatt-Gimblett, Barbara. 1998. *Destination Culture: Tourism, Museums, and Heritage*, Berkeley: University of California Press.

Massey, Doreen. 1995. "Places and Their Pasts." *History Workshop Journal*, no. 39 (June): 182–92. http://www.jstor.org/stable/4289361.

Medical Superintendent's Monthly Reports, Devon Record Office, March & April 1944.

Munjeri, Dawson. 2004. "Tangible and Intangible Heritage: From Difference to Convergence." *Museum International* 56 (1–2): 12–20. https://doi.org/10.1111/j.1350-0775.2004.00453.x.

Rawlinson, Kathleen. N.d. *Nurses' Memories of Exminster Hospital.* Exeter: Mulberry Printing.

Rothman, David J. 2001. *The Discovery of the Asylum. Social Order and Disorder in the New Republic.* New Brunswick & London: Aldine Transaction.

Ryan, Joanna, and Frank Thomas. 1980. *The Politics of Mental Handicap.* London: Penguin.

Schafer, R. Murray. 1977. *The Soundscape: Our Sonic Environment and the Turning of the World.* New York: Knopf.

Schofield, John. 2016. *Who Needs Experts?* London: Routledge. https://doi.org/10.4324/9781315547251.

Scull, Andrew. 2018. *Social Order/Mental Disorder: Anglo-American Psychiatry in Historical Perspective.* London: Routledge. https://doi.org/10.4324/9780429455988.

Smith, Graham, and Peter Jackson. 1999. "Narrating the Nation: The «imagined Community» of Ukrainians in Bradford." *Journal of Historical Geography* 25 (3): 367–87. https://doi.org/https://doi.org/10.1006/jhge.1999.0120.

Smith, Laurajane. 2006. *Uses of Heritage.* London: Routledge. https://doi.org/10.4324/9780203602263.

Smith, Laurajane. 2012. "Discourses of Heritage." *Nuevo Mundo.* https://journals.openedition.org/nuevomundo/64148 (accessed July 01, 2021).

Smith, Laurajane. 2013. "Editorial." *International Journal of Heritage Studies* 19 (4): 325–326.

Summerfield, Penny. 2004. "Culture and Composure: Creating Narratives of the Gendered Self in Oral History Interviews." *Cultural and Social History* 1 (1): 65–93. https://doi.org/10.1191/1478003804cs00050a

Thompson, Paul. 1978. The Voice of the Past: Oral History. Oxford: Oxford University Press.

UNESCO. 2003. "Convention for the Safeguarding of the Intangible Cultural Heritage." http://unesdoc.unesco.org/images//0013/001325/132540e.pdf (accessed June 17, 2021)

Warren-Findley, Jannelle. 2013. "Rethinking Heritage Theory and Practice: The US Experience." *International Journal of Heritage Studies* 19 (4): 380–383. https://doi.org/10.1080/135#27258.2012.695134

CHAPTER 3

Lillhagen Is Still Elsewhere: Approaching a Dismantled Mental Hospital

Elisabeth Punzi and Helena Lindbom

Abstract

This chapter is the result of a cooperation between Helena Lindbom, with a background as a journalist and as an inmate at some of the large and now dismantled mental hospitals in Sweden, and Elisabeth Punzi, a clinical psychologist, researcher and lecturer in social work. We share an interest in the heritage of psychiatry. This article aims to demonstrate the power of narratives, and human encounters, and we perceive narratives of patients[1] as central for remembrance, and for avoiding current oppression, abuse, and de-humanizing practices. We aim to illustrate that dismantled mental hospitals need to be approached and understood with respect to embodied memories and sensations, as the body also has a narrative to tell.

The case study by which we aim to demonstrate such an alternative approach to the heritage of psychiatry, is Lillhagen psychiatric hospital in Sweden. Instead of privileging the perspective of 'experts' in the construction of Lillhagen's heritage, we combine two highly personal accounts of memories surrounding Lillhagen with an academic exploration of Lillhagen. Our focus lies on the ways in which the place and its buildings are imbued with meaning, through the lived experience of the patients, and how their narratives can allow us to learn from the past.

The chapter begins with a presentation of Lillhagen. This is followed by Helena's narrative about her experiences of Lillhagen and other institutions, and Elisabeth's narrative, which is inspired by Helena's narrative and Elisabeth's experience of being part of psychiatry, as a professional. Thereafter, we present how we worked together, followed by the theoretical concepts about places and how they can be narrated, that guided our work. Our reflections and experiences are integrated with the presentations.

---

1 Varying terms are used for individuals who seek out, or are forced to receive, psychiatric interventions. Medical terms need to be problematised since they conceal context, power imbalances, and injustice (Burstow 2013). When we use the word patient, we describe the position of the individual in the health care system. This does not mean that we have a medicalised perspective or that we assume that there is something inherently wrong with those who were or are in the patient position.

Finally, we reflect on our joint work and present our thoughts about remembrance and how patients, researchers, clinicians, and others, might work together. We intend our perspectives to contribute to the multi-faceted remembrance of dismantled mental hospitals, as well as to humane approaches and practices in the present and in the future.

1   Lillhagen

In the 1920s, the Gothenburg Town Council decided to establish Lillhagen hospital at the farmhouse Hökälla Säteri (Göteborgs Stadsfullmäktiges Handling 1922, No: 23). In the late 1920s the construction began. Melchior Wernstedt, a professor of architecture, was chosen to plan and realise the hospital. His proposal was considered the cheapest and most rational.

Lillhagen opened officially in 1933 (partially already in 1932). By then, Lillhagen had room for 1046 patients (Stadsfullmäktige 1935). The wards soon became overcrowded, and two white tower blocks with eight floors were constructed in the late sixties and early seventies. During the last decades of the twentieth century and the beginning of the twenty-first century, Lillhagen was continuously dismantled. Until 2013, a forensic psychiatry ward remained in the buildings. All other wards had been relocated or discontinued.

The two tower blocks were demolished in 2016. A large-scale construction project has taken over the site, transforming it to a residential area named Lillhagsparken. The close proximity to nature is presented as the residential area's most salient feature, alongside the vicinity to the center of Gothenburg. Buildings are still being dismantled.

A place invokes many different sensations, states, and emotions, of discomfort or wellbeing, as it is experienced by subjective individuals (Trigg 2012). The experiences and narratives of a former patient who visits a mental hospital are not the same as the experiences and narratives of relatives, researchers, or others (concerning the importance of patients' experiences, see for example LeFrancois, Menzies, and Reaume 2013; Russo and Sweeney 2016). Since the remnants of a mental hospital (or any other building) do not have inherent meanings, they should be approached and narrated from many perspectives. Thereby, their many-layered histories and complex meanings might be illuminated. The narratives of former patients are central for understanding and presenting the heritage of psychiatry in respectful and trustworthy ways. Moreover, the sensationalism that is commonplace when former psychiatric institutions are presented (Rodéhn 2020), is counteracted if patients' narratives are central.

In the preparation of this article, we decided to focus on the meaning of places and buildings, narratives and lived experiences, and what might be learned from patients and from the past. We also decided to do fieldtrips to Lillhagen together and approach both the parks and the buildings. Thanks to Dan Hansson, janitor at the unit that owns the facilities at Lillhagen, we could enter the buildings.

During one of our fieldtrips, we visited a rehab centre, *Hökälla Green Work & Rehab,* for people who for various reasons are outside the labour market. They engage in gardening and take care of the surroundings of Lillhagen. They have done enormous work during their 12.5 years of existence. The green rehab has created an environment for all kinds of birds to thrive in the area. Over 100 species can be seen there. Among others, a rare woodpecker. This environment needs a lot of maintenance. The rehab is now being dismantled. When it closes, it remains to see if, and how, the high standard that *Hökälla Green Work & Rehab* stood for can be upheld. They also have a café, where we had a cup of coffee and spoke to the other visitors. The house, which, as far as we could tell, seems to be from the first decades of the twentieth century, is about to be demolished. It used to house the occupational therapy during the Lillhagen era. The Swedish Church, Backa parish, established the rehab. They can however no longer afford it and the City of Gothenburg refuse to take over the rehab.

Every Thursday the rehab used to arrange walks, open for everyone. On the last walk, one of us participated. One man who also participated talked about how he used to work at Lillhagen but had to quit because he found it so depressing seeing all the women who repeatedly came to receive ECT (electroconvulsive therapy) and never seemed to get any better. We learned that the rehab used to have outdoor lessons for school classes and also had a program of lectures and birdwatching for the general public. To close *Hökälla Green Work & Rehab* is a loss with wider implications than just for its members and staff. We find it disappointing that no activities that involve former patients, caregivers, or staff members have been integrated at Lillhagen as witnesses and embodiments of the history of the place and as living proof of how nature can restore health, or at least play a vital part in recovery. *Hökälla Green Work & Rehab* shows that it is possible to create respectful and humane interventions that become attractive not only for those who have a personal connection to the institution, but also for the general public.

2 Helena's Narrative

It was a delay of many years before I returned to the area of Lillhagen hospital after my many stays there during the 1990's. If I did return, I always made sure I found myself on a secure distance from the hospital. It happened that

I walked below it, on the other side of the road and the railway track that crosses the beautiful cultural landscape. Now and then, I did cast a glance at the two tower blocks, white and linked together as two twins.

All changed when I got to take care of two dogs a couple of days a week around 2014. Together with them I discovered a widespread forest outside the Lillhagen park proper. We wandered along a path alongside the eastern side of the hospital. There were benches set out and I wondered in the back of my mind who used to sit there, because few of us patients in our sedated states went so far. We went to the kiosk and back. That was about it. Sometimes, we were not allowed to go out at all.

The dogs and I went up to the former water cistern, situated on a hill. We wandered along a meandering path with a rail to hold on to. We were sur-rounded by birdsong and tranquillity. Another day, we went over an artfully made footbridge into the hospital area. When we passed the white tower blocks, I felt a quivering along my spine. I hurried past. Me and the dogs took off among the low red older brick buildings and the green lawns. Lillhagen was on its way to get undramatised in my mind. For how many years did I run along the corridors of that place in my nightmares? Ten? Maybe fifteen? Always without an exit in sight. I patted the dogs. Small-talked with them. They helped me to keep the anxiety and dread away. Next time we came to visit the area, the tower blocks were dismantled.

The white huge complex, embedded in green and shining like marble in the sunshine, was definitely gone. Lillhagen was symbolised by these blocks, about which a young patient once said that they should be blown up. I under-stood exactly what he meant. Yet I couldn't grasp at that time that maybe that comment carried a double-meaning, that it mirrored how he felt inside. Me and the dogs strolled along the pathways, in the geography I remembered, which now became more and more familiar as I revisited. It felt liberating.

I was happy these main buildings were gone, not only because they were infested with asbestos and PCB but because they constituted a custody. A custody associated with many fears. A place where I, aside from my stand-ard dose, got additional medicine: The whole heavy "artillery" of neuroleptics and sleeping-pills. Neuroleptics, which nowadays are known to have harm-ful effects. To be injected with or given these medicines meant undergoing a metamorphosis: I lost my contours. I was converted into a zombie, and lost everything that could be called an interior compass, as well as my body sensa-tions. What little dignity I had disappeared. I had already been body-searched and stripped of my identity-card, wallet, cigarettes. In the middle of it all, I was still a person with traumas. Traumas that were never made "talkable", that never were suspected or seen. No one had the strength to see, deep-buried as they were, during all these years I spent in psychiatric wards.

When the neuroleptics started to affect me, I got blurred vision. I almost crept along the sides in the corridor. I could not find my room because I could not read the numbers on the doors of the rooms. To arrive at Lillhagen was a rupture every time, with no similarity to everyday life. With it followed a kind of identity loss.

I remember an old woman in a mental hospital I was a patient at. She was like an old relic, one nurse told me. Every day she looked after the flowers. I looked at her and wondered if it was the future me I saw, slithering around with a water pitcher in her hand. I have seen so many different persons at the psychiatric hospitals I have been to. I have seen the so called catatonic schizophrenics. I have seen the young mother just minutes after she had ECT-treatment, and I was frightened that a psychiatrist would come up with the idea that I somehow needed ECT. I could see the change in her. How she had become limp, without personality. And I asked myself: Did others look at me the same way?

As a patient, you don't only become docile, you become humble: the psychiatric hospital teaches you something one can hardly learn at another place. Something that is difficult to formulate in words. Therefore, I am happy that researchers start taking account of looking at the experiences that patients have had for years, decades, and centuries at mental hospitals and the like. Surveillance. Places of shame and incarceration.

I have encountered many former Lillhagen staff members. One woman who worked there told me that she had for a long time struggled to get permission to buy a hydraulic lift for the bathtub since many patients who wanted to take a bath found it difficult to enter the bathtub. When showers were installed around 1982, especially one patient refused to shower and preferred the bathtub. A shower was too much of a modernity for some of them. Finally, she got the lift so they could lift the patients into and out of the bath. On the day it arrived they celebrated with a glass of non-alcoholic cider.

• • •

I really appreciated talking to Dan Hansson during our fieldtrip to Lillhagen. He has been working in the buildings at Lillhagen for many years. I remember his colleague, Micke, vaguely from when I was a patient. They are true bearers of knowledge of a fast disappearing heritage. We walked in the basement. Elisabeth showed me the art that former patients made there. I remembered it from my hospitalizations at Lillhagen. Especially the painted forest of birch trees. It was close to the emergency intake. I realised how much compassion and understanding Dan Hansson had while I was listening to him. It was fantastic. It was fantastic to see and feel what I couldn't see or feel when I had as high doses of neuroleptics in my body as I had back then. Not that I am entirely free of it: I have medicine in case of need. But since I have started to see a psychologist, I gain more understanding of myself. I have talked to Elisabeth of how much my psychologist means to me. And I really want to convey that the "talking cure" *is* the revolution. Not the drugs. Some patients are considered unfit for the talking cure and as I perceive it, it is mainly because they get such high doses of neuroleptics that they simply cannot talk. I have been there myself. The key is within the patient himself or herself. But to "unlock" oneself, one needs other people and the therapeutic process.

I met Elisabeth for the first time at the conference *The Material and Immaterial Heritage of Psychiatry* in the beginning of June 2019 and I got the feeling that it would be possible to tell my story. My old psychologist had retired but I had already got a new one and I felt confident. Elisabeth told me that it is important that people like me, "*the mad people*", write our own history. I was at the conference two thirds of the day, then I had to go. A video of a performance in an old hospital building was just too distressing to see. I couldn't watch it to the end. The movements the artist made, like she was in a metamorphosis, reminded me of being injected with Haldol.

• • •

To get invited to the heritage conference was amazing. The atmosphere of kindness and openness. To hear the lecturers talk about a world that I thought no one was interested in, and basically inexplicable, was even more amazing. They could give words to things I had experienced but couldn't put in language myself, couldn't communicate. Then to get a request from Elisabeth to get involved in this way was an opportunity I felt ready to grasp.

• • •

My trauma was not resolved at the hospital. It got worse as I was retraumatised the same day I arrived. What brought me to the hospital in the first place was traumatic experiences of sexual abuse during a half-year stay in Asia. One incident was when a person in a position of authority came knocking on the door to my small rented house, asking to see my passport, then telling me to come with him. That's how it happened. This was repeated for several days. No one had a clue of what I had been exposed to, and I myself had relegated it to the deep recesses of my mind. No one understood or asked. Instead, they thought I had been taking drugs and my parents thought I had become a member of a sect. And the years went by. Until I started to trust a social worker and started to talk. Now, my psychologist says that if I could have talked to someone from the start, matters would have been different.

As I started to contemplate and talk about my almost 30 years in and out of psychiatric hospitals in therapy, I have learned about myself. But that is not enough. One needs to learn about one's surroundings, the people in it, and all that makes up one's place in the world. I really learned the hard way. It was not evident in any way that I could make it. Doomed as I was by the psychiatrist as "uncurable". And there is always more to know. I am grateful for all the people who care and who strive to dig this knowledge out and share it along with their experience, or non-experience. We cannot take it for granted. And foremost I feel gratitude to those who study and try to understand trauma.

Considering my experiences, I have only one wish: To again and again underline how important it is to have someone to talk to. Someone who listens. Who has not decided on who you are beforehand. Who understands that some things are difficult to talk about. Even in one's own family. One cannot talk to just anybody. One Tibetan Guru I met believed in me when no one around me did. He challenged the view that it was something "biochemical", something that had nothing to do with what had happened to me. We are all interdependent. We need each other. It's not where you come from, but how you understand things.

I also want to write about a person who has been in my everyday life since about a year or two. She is a former hairdresser at Lillhagen. When I feel a little bit down, I can come and visit her. She gives me a cup of coffee and we chat. Sometimes we drink lemonade. She knows part of my world of experience, like few others do.

3   Elisabeth's Narrative

Throughout the work with this chapter, I have pondered my memories of Lillhagen hospital. I never worked at, was neither a patient, nor visited the hospital when it was a hospital. Yet, growing up in the surroundings of Gothenburg, Lillhagen was always in the back of my mind. I have friends who were patients at Lillhagen. Some of them are not alive anymore. Having learned more about psychiatry and its methods, including the medicines and treatments Helena describes, I have tried to grasp what my friends went through. I knew them before they were patients, knew their difficulties and distress. From my point of view, they became de-humanizsed once they were considered psychiatric patients. I can understand why some of them came to the tragic conclusion that life was meaningless. I am grateful to Helena for sharing her story with me and for contributing her trust, experiences, and time. What I have learned from Helena, I could never have learned from books, teachings, supervision, or routine research.

During my internships as a psychology student, and as a practitioner, I have visited and worked at other psychiatric hospitals. I have seen staff members who supported patients, treated them with respect and concern, approaching them for what they were: unique human beings. Most staff members I saw were average, did their job. I have also seen patients being abused and ridiculed. Once, I saw two psychiatric aides make a patient who asked for a cup of coffee in a perfectly adequate way, beg for it. They laughed and dictated what he should say. When he did, they gave him coffee. I was doing my internship. I was shocked, could not speak. I could not believe it. I went to another room, started crying, took my belongings, left the ward and never came back. I regret I did not react.

My experiences have made me question mental health care and the education nurses, psychiatric aides, psychiatrists, psychologists, researchers, and others receive. As a psychologist and researcher, I consider myself an ally to survivors and critical users. Yet, I am aware that I am also a representative of the system. My tears cannot be compared to the suffering of the patients. Moreover, practitioners become complicit with the system, in one way or another. Therefore, I do not work as a practitioner anymore. I do not have the strength to compromise with the stupidities of the organisations, the diagnostic systems and the inadequate or even abusive treatment methods.

I believe that survivors, users, practitioners, researchers, close ones, and laypersons should work together to change the system, the perceptions of mental distress, and healing. We have different experiences and perspectives and complement each other. When Helena shares her experiences of being so affected by medicine that she could not find her room, and how her sense of her body became so distorted she lost both her contours and her sense of self, I realise my own wrongdoings. Now, I understand that as a practitioner I often took the effects of medication as symptoms. My patients could describe how they lost their sense of themselves, sometimes even their sense of existing. Helena's narrative makes me realise that I contributed to pathologizing them. Throughout my many years of education and clinical practice, experiences such as Helena's were never discussed.

I really tried to support my patients and do not blame my education for my failures, but I think we need to improve the attitudes among health care practitioners, and change perspectives, also during education. We need to understand the power of listening, learn from patients, and question the expertise of the psy-disciplines. We also need to appreciate that experiences are narrated through language, creative expressions, bodily sensations, appearances, and experiences that are connected to places and the memories these places hold. To remember places of oppression is a way of recognizing those who were incarcerated there. What we preserve and how we preserve and narrate it, says something about what is valued. Narratives about the past say something about our current perceptions, which, in turn, shape current and future practices. In order to understand how to approach mental distress and in order to humanize mental health care, we need to approach the heritage of psychiatry and the narratives of patients. Together.

4 Our Work Together

During the preparation of this chapter, we took the following steps and came to the following decisions: The first step was to have multiple dialogues about our perspectives. We discussed how we perceived psychiatry, built environment (not only connected to psychiatry) as well as remembrance, heritage, and patients' narratives. We also reflected on our perceptions of mental distress, trauma, and the varying experiences and needs of patients and staff members. It was important for us to understand each other's perspectives and experiences. When we sufficiently understood each other's perspectives and had reached a shared perspective, we started to discuss theories and concepts we found interesting.

It should be acknowledged that the process was not linear and we did not decide everything in detail. Only when we started our first fieldtrip to Lillhagen, we decided how to move along with it. We decided to start with Helena showing Elisabeth around, telling what she sensed was important and that came to her mind. Helena had shared parts of her narrative with Elisabeth before the fieldtrip. Elisabeth was able to ask questions and thereby deepen her understanding of Helena's experiences, and of Lillhagen. We were able to pose questions to Dan Hansson and his colleague Micke, who had both worked at Lillhagen since the seventies. Thereby, we gained knowledge about when houses were built or dismantled and where fences and entrances had been placed. The amount of knowledge and the narratives Dan and Micke shared with us cannot, unfortunately, be represented here.

Two fieldtrips were conducted in the fall of 2019 and one was performed in spring 2020. In between the fieldtrips we immersed ourselves in literature about places, the history of psychiatry, mental distress and trauma, and non-medical approaches to mental distress and trauma. And we started writing. We wrote a lot and as the process evolved, we decided what to exclude, what to keep and what to revise. The writing process was also a way of understanding. Not all of the literature we read is referred in this text, but it was important for us to read a lot in order to gain a shared understanding of perspectives, concepts, and theories. Moreover, through reading fiction and poetry, we became inspired and also understood the influence of popular culture on how mental distress and patients are perceived, for better and for worse. Kate Zambreno's (2014) book about female authors who were also psychiatric patients became a basis for reflections. Zambreno for example describes how Zelda Fitzgerald, unappreciated as a writer in her lifetime, died in a fire in the mental hospital where she was hospitalised. The movie and the book *One Flew Over the Cuckoo's Nest* (Kesey 1963) also was a point of reference for our reflections on how to approach dismantled hospitals. These books portray the past but from different perspectives. We truly appreciate *One Flew Over the Cuckoo's Nest* and simultaneously it needs to be noted that it represents a male perspective; the women are bad mothers, bad nurses, or prostitutes. Zambreno portrays women who strived to find their voices and express themselves which was inspiring for us.

We wanted to permit emotions and processes to be represented in the text. This might give the chapter a somewhat scattered impression. Nevertheless, this way of writing enhances the possibility to challenge conventional medically oriented narratives of psychiatry (Eivergård and Jönsson 2005), exemplify how patients and researchers can work together, and examine the importance of places, narratives and human encounters.

5   Places, Meanings and Narratives

Remembrance of places where abuse and oppression occurred is important, not least since they invoke embodied emotions and memories that inform our understanding of the place and of the individuals who experienced it (Steele, Djuric, Hibberd, and Yeh 2020; Trigg 2012). The experience of a place is also influenced by expectations, intentions, knowledge, and habitus of the individual who encounters it (Frykman 2012). We need to acknowledge that the place and its buildings influence our life-world, and at the same time our life-world influences the sites we encounter (Frykman 2012, 64). In the example of mental hospitals, they might be presented as healing environments, embedded in therapeutic landscapes, and simultaneously as haunted places, invoking images of horror (Punzi 2019; Yahm 2014).

Following Trigg (2012) and Frykman (2012), we argue that patients' opportunities to bear witness are enhanced by the very places in which oppression occurred. The body remembers, the body narrates. Helena's memories of losing her contours, groping her way through the corridors of Lillhagen is a defining example of how places evoke memories that support others', including Elisabeth's, understanding of what it means to be a psychiatric patient.

Efforts to create so-called therapeutic environments appear to come in cycles. It should however be noted that ideas of so-called therapeutic environments are rarely based on experiences of patients or staff members, but rather represent ideas of stakeholders and architects who have the power to pursue their agendas and have something to win from establishing these spaces (Punzi 2018). Places reproduce hegemony and power even though they are presented as innocent (Dion 2012). We therefore argue that the renewed interest in hospital design needs to be problematised and critically examined.

We also argue that it is necessary to critically examine the tendency to transform former mental hospitals into attractive and often expensive residential areas that exploit the past through highlighting the beauty of the buildings and the proximity to nature. This tendency excludes the narratives of patients and the fact that beauty cannot mitigate the embodied and place-based experience of abuse and oppression and that the place might also be a meaningful part of remembrance and of patients' narratives that hold keys to supportive relationships, such as Helena's relationship with the hairdresser. Ironically, the rising property prices as well our argument shows the importance of these sites and their buildings.

The differing views concerning Lillhagen and its past become apparent through the construction work at the site. Under the headline *"Lillhagen söker nya boende"* (Lillhagen searching new inhabitants) the local paper *GöteborgDi-rekt* (Mia Petterson) cites the vice chairman of *Byggnadsnämnden* (the Building Committee of the City of Gothenburg) who says that people no longer associate Lillhagen *"as they used to"*, with its past. Nevertheless, the article stresses that the citizens still associate Lillhagen with *"psychiatric care"*. The chief executive of the construction company, Sören Gustafsson, says that he would have preferred the old name Hökälla, and had some doubts about the new name, *Lillhagsparken*.

We ask ourselves why former patients or patient organisations were not included in the process or in the article. Neither the politician, nor the chief executive, seem to consider the possibility to acknowledge the place as a heritage of psychiatry and of former patients. Maybe they assume that people do not want to be reminded of the history. We assume that people, at least some, actually might have a genuine interest and may want to understand and may want to listen to and understand patients' narratives. After all, many people have their own experiences of mental distress or have people close to them with such experiences. It is reasonable to think that they would like to recognise the heritage of psychiatry and the narratives of the patients.

Arguments about dark histories that should be forgotten tend to surface when economic interests are at stake (Eivergård and Jönsson 2005). By the turn of the century, The City of Gothenburg's property managers of Lillhagen expressed that the small hospital museum that by then was situated at the site "should be a resource, as a meeting place for those who are interested in the history and cultural heritage of the area" (Eivergård and Jönsson 2005). The museum at the site was discontinued and became integrated in *Medicinhistoriska Museet* (Museum of Medical History), Gothenburg. We ask ourselves how the change in perspective and the view of Lillhagen's heritage occurred and why. We dare to guess that it has something to do with money.

It should be noted that *Medicinhistoriska Museet* dedicates a considerable part of their exhibition to psychiatry and avoids presenting psychiatry as a story of medical success and rather emphasises the milieus and the patients' perspectives (Eivergård and Jönsson 2005). It should also be noted that in the case of Lillhagen, former employees have predominantly shown an interest in the fate of the place, and have argued for remembrance. We want to acknowledge Dan and Micke who helped us to enter the buildings, and also Christer (who previously worked at Lillhagen) and Lisa and Annica who work at *Medicinhistoriska*. They show a genuine interest in narrating the heritage of Lillhagen and in the experiences of the patients. At least the patients' voices are represented in some form, albeit through the museum or through the narratives of Dan and Micke. In most cases, the voices of the patients are not heard at all.

Yahm (2014) describes that the *Oregon State Hospital Museum of Mental Health*, established in the hospital buildings that were the setting for the movie *One Flew Over the Cuckoo's Nest*, capitalises on its history and simultaneously tries to distance itself from it, for example though avoiding narratives of control. Focus is, as often, on medical history (Coleborne 2003; LeFrancois, Menzies, and Reaume 2013). According to Yahm (2014), users have been involved in the presentations, and the museum strives to present a user perspective: nevertheless, the narrative about the hospital does not represent a user perspective. It should be noted that a former patient might see a movie like *One Flew Over the Cuckoos' Nest* as part of the anti-psychiatry movement or as a description of oppression and abuse. To others, the movie might be understood as a metaphor for society as large. At *Oregon State Hospital Museum of Mental Health*, the movie becomes such a metaphor. Visitors encounter signs asking *Who is the Big Nurse in Your Life*? We think it might be relevant to present psychiatric oppression as a metaphor, if it is made explicit that psychiatry is also about real deeds that people have been exposed to. If psychiatric oppression becomes a metaphor, confrontation with oppression and control, currently and throughout the history of psychiatry, however are avoided (Yahm 2014). People who have been controlled, oppressed, and abused become misrecognised when the oppressive history is diluted. Paradoxically, there is often a simultaneous tendency to exhibit historical horror and abuse. This is sometimes fuelled by sensationalism, exploitation, or by attempts to portray psychiatry as a story of medical success and progress (Beitik 2012; Conroy and Downey 2020). Presentations of medical success give the impression that nothing is wrong with psychiatry as a discipline. Violent interventions and oppression, such as lobotomy and physical punishment, are presented as past mistakes, but we do not need to question current practices or perspectives, or psychiatry as a discipline.

Accordingly, remembrance is important for correcting misrepresentations of history and for recognizing patients as individuals and as a collective. Reaume in his research on the asylum on Queen Street in Toronto (see chapter by Reaume in this volume) shows that patients were used as unpaid laborers. This included building and repairing many of the structures behind which they were confined, including still existing walls of this property (Reaume 2016). By stressing that these walls were built by patients, not as part of therapy but as forced labour, Reaume writes a counter history and shows how patients actually were capable, but their capabilities were exploited. This counter history and the efforts of the Psychiatric Survivor Archives of Toronto resulted in public plaques commemorating the labour of psychiatric patients being installed at the site. This was supported by representatives of the hospital that currently operates on the site and by the wider mad and local community (Reaume 2016). This supports our assumption that the community surrounding Lillhagen might actually be interested in the heritage of the site. Reaume engages in processes of counter-mapping that allow minority groups to challenge some of the 'taken of granteds' of heritage management, and encourages people to celebrate their everyday experiences (Harrison 2011, 91).

Before we present our final reflections and give some suggestions, we would like to provide a place-based experience, shared by Helena.

• • •

– Are you afraid?
I nod.
– You can hold my hand if you want to.

Gratefully, I hold the hand. It holds me firmly. I sit quietly in the taxi on the way to Lillhagen.

There is no fence surrounding Lillhagen, no gate-keeper we need to pass. The fence probably disappeared in the nineties (Nordlund 2014, 22). This must have been in the early nineties. I don't remember.

The taxi drives behind the tower buildings. I am amazed. I have never seen the buildings from this side. The hospital area is so much bigger than I thought, and yet, a place not only defined by its spatial expansion. As Malpas (2007, 48) writes; *"place" 'should not be understood as referring primarily to the idea that in which an entity is located or positioned."* Lillhagen is a specific site. But it is also elsewhere. Extends its geographical and architectural features.

The psychiatric aide hands me over to the ward. Something is happening. Another patient is violent. They ask me to wait, locked in an adjoining room. Anxiety increases again. Terrified, I wonder what happens. Then, I am allocated to a room. Receive sleeping pills and other medicines. Try to relax and fall asleep. I wish I had a radio I could listen to before I fall asleep. To mitigate the thoughts. Be accompanied by the radio voice. Avoid the sounds from the ward. To arrive at a ward always gives a feeling of reaching an end station: I do not know what happens next. The multitude of medicines strikes like a bomb and makes me lose the thread. I am in some kind of limbo.

To find the threads again, after a long life in and out of psychiatric hospitals is hard work. In a way, a detective work, a puzzle. Sometimes I glimpse something. Something that wants to say something.

I experienced such a glimpse during one of my many walks at Lillhagen. Or maybe I was at home, looking at photos I have taken of the tower buildings before they were dismantled. Now I know one reason why they seemed so terrifying to me. They resemble the tower block me and family lived in the year before we moved to the countryside. Through this connection, which I discussed with Elisabeth, some memories became clearer, specifically the summer I spent alone with my mother when I had chicken-pox and couldn't accompany my siblings to my grandparents. I began first class there, and I think I was in school for a month there, before we moved and the family was reunited. When the memories became clearer, I could start talking about this in psychotherapy. It had been so frightening; I could not admit the feelings it caused. But there is always an alarm-clock ringing somewhere. Sooner or later one has to listen to it again. In my case it was a neighbour girl. She cut my hair and it was my first loss of identity. She asked if she could cut my hair.

– Are you able to cut hair?

– Yes, she said, with the confidence of a seven-year-old.

I let her do it. She cut my hair short. Large, rough cuts.

When I came home, I looked at myself in the mirror. I was in shock, despair. I do not remember if I cried but I experienced a loss of identity. I didn't go outside for three days. Finally, my mother could sneak me out and take me to a hairdresser she knew in the countryside who could adjust it. I didn't want to expose myself to anyone. It was an identity crisis. I did not want to look like a boy and I was ashamed I had not trusted my own feelings and refused the haircut.

I also remember the large windows and magnificent view at Lillhagen. Drawn to the windows, I looked at the scenery and life outside the building. Even though I was aware that I never fully could take in the scenery, appreciate it, or experience the feeling, I am sure I benefited from it. Nevertheless, being outdoors is good for one's health and we seem to live too much of our lives indoors (Li 2018). Our physical intelligence, also named embodied cognition, becomes inactive when we are not physically engaged (Grafton 2020, 7). As Grafton points out, if you want to learn the feel of slipping tires, your hands have to be on the wheel of the car. If you want to detect the tipsiness of a ladder your feet need to be balanced on it. You also need to devote time and energy: texting, virtual goggles, reading, and rationalizing won't get the job done, Grafton emphasises (*ibid.*).

When incarcerated, you lose your physical intelligence. As a patient, one intuitively senses this when one is admitted to the hospital. This is not talked about, the body is not really acknowledged. Grafton sees physical intelligence as a fundamental kind of knowing (*ibid.*, 9). Being medicated and taken out of your everyday environment makes something to you that includes the body and its ways of knowing.

The power of 'nature' has long been acknowledged and remains central within ongoing research identifying benefits of interactions with woodlands, parks and gardens, not least for young people (Milligan and Bingley 2007) and people who experience mental distress (Adams and Morgan 2018). As a society, we must increase the possibilities for holistic healing, create a system that is attuned to the patients' needs.

I remember an evening when me and another patient asked for "fika"[2] and the staff members just shook their heads. There is no evening-fika, they said. It has been cut down. Costs should be reduced. The staff members retire to the office. The whole staff is there. Talking, perhaps about their future and the future of Lillhagen. The ward is abandoned. We are left to interpret the signs,

---

2   "Fika" could be translated to coffee break but such a translation would miss the meaning of "fika". Fika is more than a coffee break; it signifies a social meeting that means to socialise, chat, and have coffee, sandwiches and cookies.

grasp what is going on. The atmosphere has changed. Gloomy. In the bathroom with its many cubicles there is wet paper on the floor, it is untidy and messy. It hits me that the dismantling of the interior started long before the actual dismantling of the buildings.

6　　Final Reflections and Some Suggestions

To understand the heritage and places of psychiatry, one needs to understand one's own position and approach. For Helena it became important to search the archives to find facts and narratives. For Elisabeth it became important to see how the heritage of psychiatry has been approached internationally. We believe we complement each other.

Costa et al. (2012) write that patients' narratives are opportunities to learn, if they are seen as counter narratives with potentials for change, and do not become forms of entertainment, sensationalism, or exploitation. There is a risk that patients' narratives become coopted, which means that patients are invited to tell their narratives as long as they are not too critical, whereby the institution concerned can pride itself of having involved users (Eriksson 2013).

Hopefully, we have shown a possible way to learn from each other and create a form of mutual counter narrative. Helena expresses it with the following words: "This is something Elisabeth has emphasised, and she emphasised the importance of one's own history. That this is so self-evident and natural for her strengthens my belief in what I do, that it is not something vain or nostalgic in a denigrating way." In Elisabeth's words: "To do this together, and engage in a process we did not know exactly where it would lead ... Sometimes I doubted the process and asked Helena if we should discontinue but she motivated me to pursue. I am also happy that we decided to make the process explicit. This is meaningful and honest, but rarely done in academia."

Nostalgia, once deemed an illness, has undergone a transformation and the concept now also has a positive connotation, since thinking about and appreciating the past enhances a sense of meaning (Routledge et al. 2011). We hope our work exemplifies that as human beings, we form relationships to places where significant events have occurred and where emotions have been central. We have also shown how places and building become superimposed on one another. Where does the tower building from childhood end and where does the tower buildings of Lillhagen begin?

Moreover, we sense that terrifying experiences should not be perceived as signs of disorders. They are part of personal narratives. Frightening, overwhelming and sometimes complicating for everyday life, but understandable, and with narrative threads. In Helena's narrative there is a thread connecting the tower buildings. There is also a narrative thread between the childhood countryside, the love for nature and the arguments for humane care that involves nature, gardening, and animals. And coffee is important. We both remember significant events connected to coffee. And when we had coffee at *Green Rehab* we could talk to people and get to know the place. There is also a connection between the meaningful relationship to the hairdresser from Lillhagen and the childhood haircut. Elisabeth has a similar experience. As a child, her friend cut her hair. It looked, and felt terrible. She recognises herself when Helena expresses the shame of not trusting her own feelings. Together we talked about how such an ordinary event as a haircut could be loaded with meaning. When we were at Lillhagen, Helena showed Elisabeth where the hair salon was. It is important as a place, as a memory and as part of the narrative we are presenting and constructing together.

Finally, we would like to reflect on our mutual process and give some suggestions on how to work together. Firstly, we find it important to have plenty of time. This enhances the possibilities to understand each other's perspectives, read, write, and rewrite. We have rewritten this text many, many times and have decided to continue writing together. We created a document in which we saved parts of our text that were outside the scope of this article, parts that we sensed were important and we perhaps would want to return to. We recommend others to do the same, since this counteracts a sense of stress. It is not now or never. This is what we do right now. Later on, we can write about other topics. Plenty of time also reassures the possibility to change one's mind. One can reflect on choice of words and what one wants to share, or keep to oneself. Not telling everything is not about fear or shame, it is about personal integrity and respect for others.

Secondly, we find it important to pose questions such as the following: What is important for oneself and what does one wish to forget? What is needed for healing? This is maybe specifically important for writers with lived experience, since it is challenging and overwhelming to investigate one's history and put words to it. With Helena's words:

> Without Elisabeth I would not have gone so deep, but I am happy I did, even though I sometimes was overwhelmed by emotions, had taken in a bit too much, too soon. It is difficult to sort my feelings out, to sense what I really feel and what it represents and means to me. It's important to have time to breathe, and reflect over what I have read and how it connects to the society we live in. Me, and many others, need a safe place within ourselves in order take in everything. It is ongoing work.

Writing could be a safe place, a room for those who have none (Tygstrup 2008). Through writing, one might investigate what is important to forget and remember, and how healing can develop. Nostalgia is important for existential well-being (Routledge et al. 2011). Difficulties connected to places cannot however only be a question of nostalgia. As witnesses and subjects, we have a duty to find a place in the world, to write ourselves a place. This is in line with Robertson's perspective on heritage: "Heritage thinking, like heritage management cannot be solely top-down; we need to listen to local voices expressing 'heritage from below' and their claim to heritage rights" (Robertson 2012, 20, cited in Logan, Craith, and Kockel 2015).

Thirdly, we encourage others to explore places and be physically involved in their investigations. Life is physical and social. Social and material needs, and sense of connectedness should not be devalued (Cummins 2019) and we need to acknowledge the importance of meaningful activities and relationships, they constitute a social cure (Jetten et al. 2019). We specifically talked about the impact of reading and writing, and of nature. And we engaged with nature. Our walks were not only informative; they were beautiful, and we had a great time. Beauty and joy should not be overlooked. Moreover, the possible obstacles of mutual writing, and the need for specific recommendations for academics/practitioners and users/survivors writing together, should not be exaggerated. After all, writing is rewarding but is also a process that is sometimes demanding, sometimes forces one to exclude parts that one finds important. It is often challenging to write together, even for persons with a shared background. Many academic collaborations have collapsed because of difficulties during the writing process. Maybe, the suggestions we have provided are not so much suggestion to researchers and patients writing together as they are to anyone writing together. Maybe that sounded a bit grandiose for us to express, but still …

· · ·

We have focused on the possibilities to learn from the past. Yet, psychiatry seems paralyzed, cannot change and see that diagnoses and medicines are no solutions. Nature, along with the social cure and the talking cure are parts of the heritage of psychiatry, yet their possibilities are not taken seriously. A new physical and relational environment is needed; calm and with a sense of security which is a prerequisite for opening up as a patient, confide, and get listened to. Maybe in a clearing in a forest. The talking cure usually takes place once or twice a week, 45 or 50 minutes. The rest of the time, one needs to be in a non-threatening environment, an environment one can lean against, rest in. Such places must be actively sought out and created. Lillhagen is a beautiful place. But we need to ask, who has access to the beauty? It remains to see how accessible to the public *Lillhagsparken* will be. There is always a risk that former institutions get sucked up by commercial interests, perhaps rebuilt as "gated communities", keeping trespassers out.

After the establishments, transformations, and dismantlings, Lillhagen is still elsewhere. The narratives of experience, the "final words" from those who really made up Lillhagen, the patients, are still lacking. Those voices are underrepresented (see Nordlund 2016, 9, 36) and have yet to take form and bear witness. There is always something more to know, there are always experiences that are still elsewhere. Still yearning to be asked for, and narrated.

References

Adams, Matthew, and Julie Morgan. 2018. "Mental Health Recovery and Nature: How Social and Personal Dynamics are Important." *Ecopsychology* 10 (1): 44–52.

Beitik, E. S. 2012. "The Ghosts of Institutionalization at Pennhurst's Haunted Asylum." *Hastings Center Report* 42: 22–24.

Coleborne, Catharine. 2003. "Remembering Psychiatry's Past. The Psychiatric Collection and Its display at Porirua Hospital Museum, New Zealand." *Journal of Material Culture* 8: 97–118.

Costa, Lucy, Jijian Voronka, Danielle Landry, Jenna Reid, Becky McFarlane, David Reville, and Kathryn Church. 2012. "Recovering our Stories: A Small Act of Resistance." *Studies in Social Justice* 6: 85–101.

Dion, Nicholas. 2012. *Spacing Freud: Space and Place in Psychoanalytic Theory*. PhD diss., University of Toronto.

Downey, Dennis B., and James W. Conroy. 2020. *Pennhurst and Struggle for Disability Rights*. Pennsylvania: Keystone Books.

Eivergård, M., and L.-E. Jönsson. 2005. *Sinnesjukhus som kulturarv*. [Mental Hospitals as Cultural Heritage.] Report. Stockholm: Riksantikvarieämbetet.

Eriksson, Erik. 2013. "To Tell the Right Story: Functions of the Personal User Narrative in Service User Involvement." *Journal of Comparative Social Work* 2: 2–32.

Frykman, Jonas. 2012. *Berörd. Plats, kropp och ting i fenomenologisk kulturanalys*. [Touched. Place, body and object in phenomenological culture analysis]. Stockholm: Carlsson.

Grafton, Scott. 2020. *Physical Intelligence. The Science of Uniting Mind and Body*. London: John Murray Publishers.

Harrison, Rodney. 2011. "'Counter Mapping' Heritage, Communities and Places in Australia and the UK." In *Local Heritage, Global Context. Cultural Perspectives on Sense of Place,* edited by John Shoefield and Rosy Szymanski, 79–98. Farnham: Ashgate.

Jetten, Jolanda, S. Alexander Haskam, Tegan Cruwys, Katharine Greenaway, Catherine Haslam, and Niklas K. Steffens. 2017. "Advancing the Social Identity Approach to Health and Well-Being: Processing the Social Cure Research Agenda." *European Journal of Social Psychology* 47: 789–802.

Kesey, Ken. 1963. *One Flew Over the Cuckoo's Nest.* New York: Berkley.

LeFrancois, Brenda. A., Robert Menzies, and Geoffrey Reaume, ed. 2013. *Mad Matters. A Critical Reader in Canadian Mad Studies.* Toronto: Canadian Scholars' Press.

Li, Qing. 2018. *Forest Bathing: How Trees Can Help You Find Health and Happiness.* New York: Viking.

Logan, William, Máiréad Nic Craith, and Ullrich Kockel, ed. 2015. *Companion to Heritage Studies.* Sussex: Wiley Blackwell.

Malpas, Jeff. 2006. *Heidegger's Topology. Being, Place, World.* Boston: MIT Press.

Milligan, Christine, and Amanda Bingley. 2007. "Restoratives Places of Scary Spaces? The Impact of Woodland on the Mental Well-Being of Young Adults." *Health & Place* 13: 799–811.

Nordlund, Cecilia. 2014. *Lillhagens sjukhus som immateriellt kulturarv – bärare av före detta patienters minnen och berättelser.* [Lillhagen hospital as immaterial heritage – bearer of former patinets and narratives.] Bachelor thesis. Institutionen för kulturvård [Department of Conservation]. Gothenburg University.

Punzi, Elisabeth. 2018. "Brave New Psychiatry and the Idealization of Nonplaces: A Critical Discourse Analysis." *Ethical Human Psychology and Psychiatry* 20: 100–112.

Punzi, Elisabeth. 2019. "Ghost Walks or Thoughtful Remembrance. How Should the Heritage of Psychiatry be Approached?" *Journal of Critical Psychology, Counselling and Psychotherapy* 19: 242–251.

Reaume, Geoffrey. 2016. "A Wall's Heritage: Making Mad People's History Public." *Public Disability History* 1, 20.

Robertson, Iain. J. M. 2012. *Heritage from Below.* Farnham: Ashgate.

Rodéhn, Cecilia. 2020. "Emotions in the Museum of Medicine. An Investigation of How Museum Educators Employ Emotions and What these Emotions do." *International Journal of Heritage Studies* 26: 201–213.

Routledge, Clay, Jamie Arndt, Tim Wildschut, Constantine Sedikides, Claire Hart, Jacob Juhl, J.J.M. Vingerhoets, and Wolff Schlotz. 2011. "The Past Makes the Present Meaningful: Nostalgia as an Existential Resource." *Journal of Personality and Social Psychology* 101: 638–652.

Russo, Jane, and Angela Sweeney. 2016. *Searching for a Rose Garden. Challenging Psychiatry, Fostering Mad Studies.* Monmouth: PCCS.

Steele, Linda, Bonney Djuric, Lily Hibberd, and Fiona Yeh. 2020. "Parramatta Female Factory Precinct as a Site of Conscience: Using Institutional Pasts to Shape Just Legal Futures." *The University of New South Wales Law Journal*, in press.

Trigg, Dylan. 2012. *The Memory of Place. A Phenomenology of the Uncanny*. Athens: Ohio University Press.

Tygstrup, Frederik. 2008. "Livets rum, erindringens form. W. G. Sebalds Austerlitz og vidnesbyrdlitteraturen." [Rooms of life, the form of memories. W. G. Sebald's Austerlitz and witness literature]. *Passage* 58: 97–116.

Yahm, Sarah. 2014. "Oregon State Hospital of Mental Health. (Critical essay)." *The Journal of American History* 101: 203–208.

Zambreno, Kate. 2014. *Heroines*. New York: Harper Perennial.

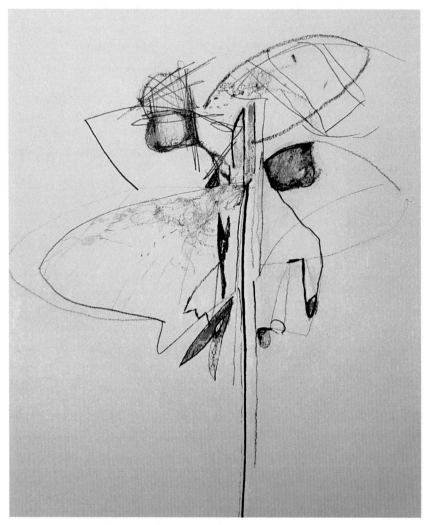

FIGURE 3.1   Marta Wandt

CHAPTER 4

Narratives of De-Institutionalisation: Patient and Community Responses to Mental Hospital Closures in England

Rob Ellis and Rob Light

Abstract

This chapter uses a previously untapped archive of oral histories, collected at a mental hospital in the north of England in the 1980s. Its aim is to broaden our understanding of life and work within it, and to consider the narratives that emerged at a time when it was earmarked for closure. The oral history archive documents the hopes and fears of patients as their hospital and, often, their home was slowly closed down around them. The chapter considers the questions being asked of the participants and explores the factors that shaped their development. It also contrasts them with the local community's responses to the hospital's closure and the deinstitutionalisation of its patients. By engaging with the longer-term history of the hospital and its community relations, this chapter builds on recent research which has placed patient narratives at the heart of what was a pivotal period in mental health care provision, with a view to providing a more representative picture of the impact it had on those affected.

Keywords

community care – deinstitutionalisation – patients – testimony – Storthes Hall – 1980s

1   Introduction

In 1985, in the north of England, Douglas Spencer, the Medical Director of the Meanwood Park Hospital and Lecturer in Psychiatry at the University of Leeds, wrote a short history of Storthes Hall Hospital. A large in-patient mental facility that had begun life as the West Riding Asylum in nearby Huddersfield, it had been scheduled for closure and, as a keen amateur historian, Spencer wanted to "preserve information about the hospital before it was lost forever" (Spencer 1985). There was nothing particularly novel about his desire to record the past histories of psychiatric endeavour (Coleborne and MacKinnon 2011) and in many ways the notes he made were uncontroversial, touching only on the development of the hospital site. Elsewhere, however, he called for the establishment of a national museum of psychiatry for the UK, and this prompted discussion within the field about what its focus might be (Ellis 2015, 332). Already feeling embattled by the scaling back of in-patient services and media reports of scandalous treatment of vulnerable individuals, the discipline of psychiatry was also under attack from a new breed of social historian. Their new revisionist histories challenged the previously benign narratives of psychiatry and institutional care that had often been written by those who worked in the sector. There were fears in some quarters that the opening up of archival material from former institutions would only lead to more negative analyses and interpretations.

There can be little doubt that this battle over the narrative accounts of psychiatry's past was framed by the forces of deinstitutionalisation and the shifting nature of treatment regimes around the globe. Indeed, to the casual observer, the closure of large hospitals, such as Storthes Hall, appears to mark a neat point of departure but its longer-term history is messy and sometimes obscure. While some historians point to the 1950s as the decade in which the theoretical and physical dismantling of institutional paradigms began, others have sought to uncover the longer-term trajectory of institutional and extra-institutional options in what is often known as the mixed economy of care. In the UK at least, in-patient numbers had fallen significantly by the 1970s but it was not until the 1980s that a policy of closure was "pursued aggressively [...] with most hospitals actually closing in the 1990s." (Bartlett and Sandland 2007, 63; Crossley 2006, 57; Taylor 2015, 118–119) On the face of it, the will to close large-scale mental institutions and instigate a policy of "community care" looks progressive, but this has been further complicated by studies which have unpacked the motivations of politicians and policy makers. The result has been a complex picture in which economic determinist arguments have been contrasted with the evolution of mental health care and treatments that appeared to facilitate the change (Crossley 2006, 57–58; Rafferty 1996, 26; Gallagher 2018, 3).

Equally, the move to community care was initially welcomed by service user groups and survivor networks (Payne 1999, 244–245) but longer-term assessments of its impact, in some cases, have been damning. Central to this has been its funding (Payne 1999, 244–245) and opposition Members of Parliament [MPs] described its ill-defined and under-resourced nature as a "catastrophe", while Barbara Taylor, a historian and former mental hospital in-patient, labelled the shifting emphasis a "debacle" (Taylor 2015, 118–119). Writing in 1991,

Baroness Elaine Murphy, another historian and mental health campaigner, categorised the period from 1962–1990 as community care's "Disaster Years" (quoted in Taylor 2015, 118–119) and, as Nick Crossley notes, by the end of the 1990s, "even the government was calling community care a failure" (Crossley 2006, 66). Moreover, it is important to recognise that the closure of large mental hospitals has not led to the end of institutionalisation in some forms. Numbers of in-patient admissions remain significantly high, albeit with shorter average lengths of stay and, since the 1990s, there has been an increase in the number of compulsory detentions (Turner, Hayward, Angel, et al., 604–605; Rafferty 1996, 26).

Nevertheless, the closure of large-scale former mental hospitals has prompted a fascination with their histories. A number of public history projects have sought to remember these places and the things that happened in them and offer their closure as a totemic point of reference. (Memories of St David's Hospital 2020; Remembering the Mental Hospital 2020; Julich, Widlmalm 2019; Michigan Radio 2020; Glenside Hospital Museum 2020; Craze 2014; Testimony 2020). At the same time, academic engagement with personal testimonies from patients and staff at mental hospitals has provided a complex overview of care based on multiple and sometimes competing narratives (Davies 2001; Parr, Philo, and Burns 2003; Beckman, Nelson, and Labode 2020; McCrae and Nolan 2016). In her study of Severalls Hospital, for example, Diana Gittins concluded that "contradictions abound", cautioning against a historical narrative that simply romanticised its past, or demonised it (Gittins 1998, 223). For her study Gittins conducted interviews with 65 people who had lived and worked at Severalls at different points in time, shortly before the hospital closed in 1997.

This chapter also uses oral testimonies and draws on the Pennine Heritage Oral Archive [PHOA] which includes the recollections of patients and staff at Storthes Hall. Unlike many oral histories, which were collected in the 1990s and after hospitals closed, this project began in 1984, a year before Spencer's historical essay and right at the heart of when closure programmes were being "pursued aggressively" by the British Government (Storthes Hall Oral History Recordings 1986–1988). In total, 75 interviews were conducted during the project, creating an archive which offers rare insights into how patients and staff viewed their time at the hospital and, crucially, how they saw the prospects of its closure. Using examples from this previously overlooked resource, we draw on our experiences as a historian of mental ill-health on the one hand and an oral historian on the other to explore how narratives of treatment and care were informed by historical understandings of mental hospitals and asylums, as well as the processes of deinstitutionalisation.

In particular, we consider the memories within the PHOA, and compare and contrast them with the narratives emanating from official reports and other sources. Our aim is to build on the attempts by historians and others to consider the tensions between patients and practitioners, especially where the former are "erased" from medical case notes (Porter 1985; Aaslestad 2009). Importantly, we do not claim that our approach is a scientific one and our lack of involvement in the interview process might be seen as a methodological weakness, but the opportunity to revisit historical interviews such as these "with new perceptions, possibly better informed and certainly with the benefit of additional contributory data sources" can lead to new interpretations which add value to the historical discourse (Bornat 2005). In this case, placing patient narratives at the heart of our historical analysis might uncover a more rounded understanding of the issues faced by those on the sharp end of mental health policy and practise (Coleborne 2020).

Thus, the aim here is to highlight the existence of these multiple and disparate narratives and broaden the historical discourse to provide a more representative view of the past. The first section of this chapter provides an overview of Storthes Hall's history using the available archival documents, political debates and newspaper articles. This will provide a benchmark narrative of the hospital from which we will compare and contrast the memories of staff and patients recorded in the PHOA. The second section includes an overview of the origins on the PHOA and the factors that shaped its outcomes. In addition, it briefly explains how the distinctive methodological approach of oral history offers ways to unlock individual and collective memory, and how it can provide contrasting perspectives and discursive views of institutional care and deinstitutionalisation. The following sections focus more closely on the oral history interviews in the PHOA and include patient and staff memories of their first impressions of Storthes Hall, their experiences of the hospital, and their thoughts on the prospects for its closure. To preserve the anonymity of patients, they are referred to by their first names only. Ultimately, we argue that while the narratives in the PHOA were framed by the hospital's planned closure, longer-term community (mis)understandings of what in-patient provision represented remained pervasive and influential.

2   Storthes Hall Hospital and Its History

Aside from Spencer's work little has been written about the history of Storthes Hall (Littlewood 2003; Brumby 2015; Thurgood 2008, 2010). Using extant archival resources, however, it is possible to recreate a narrative that speaks very much to the stereotypical image of mental hospitals as isolated and distant. Taking its name from the Storthes Hall mansion that had been built and owned by a local textile magnate, it opened on a former country estate in 1904. Agreeing where the new asylum was to be situated had taken almost two years of negotiations between landowners, elected members of the local county council, and local Poor Law Guardians, some of whom objected to the site. (Asylums Committee Minute Book 1897–1899). One member of the West Riding County Council complained that the site had too much woodland for an asylum. (Asylums Committee Minute Book 1897–1899). Nevertheless, just as the grand houses of polite society were separated from the rest of the world by a "sea of turf" and an encircling belt of trees (Crang 1998, 35), so too was the new asylum hidden from the nearby village of Kirkburton. Further in the distance was the town of Huddersfield, which was ten kilometres away and, although there were debates in medical and political circles about its efficacy, this spatial separation followed tropes that had been apparent for almost one hundred years.

These were not the only mental institutions in the UK but the first "County" Asylums had been built following the passing of the 1808 County Asylums Act which enabled Justices of the Peace (magistrates) in England and Wales to raise local taxes to build them. The Lunatics Act of 1845 made their building compulsory and when Storthes Hall opened, it was the 88th such institution to be built in England and Wales, and a fifth for the northern English county of Yorkshire (Fifty-ninth Report of the Commissioners in Lunacy 1905, 17). By this time, the 1888 Local Government Act meant that the management of the institutions had passed from the magistrates to an elected group of Councillors (Ellis 2020) but its geographical reach remained the same. With its catchment area covering the whole county, this was not a "local" hospital but one that was part of a wider regional network and, like other institutions in this period, it was huge.

Mirroring the demand for its services, initial plans envisaged an overall patient population of 2,250 (Storthes Hall Asylum Minute book 1898–1904, 2 Dec 1898). Almost immediately, however, admissions procedures meant that it was overcrowded. The need for in-patient beds was such that admissions began on a piecemeal basis as individual wards and facilities were completed. Within a year, a laundry room was being used to temporarily house male patients and, once all the new buildings were completed, things did not improve (Storthes Hall Asylum Minute book 1904–1906, 9 Nov 1905). In 1948, the management of Storthes Hall passed into the hands of the National Health Service [NHS] and by that time its average patient population had swelled to 3,015 (Storthes Hall Group Hospital Management Committee Reports and Statistical Tables 1948).

While official reports spoke of the cheerfulness of staff and the lack of complaints from patients on the issue of detention, there were practical problems that must have impacted on both. During this time, the ability to attract staff was a recurring issue with the establishment said to be short of 36 male and 155 female staff in 1948 (Storthes Hall Group Hospital Management Committee Reports and Statistical Tables 1949). In 1961, the staff to patient ratio at the hospital was 1:10 when the Ministry of Health's aspirations were 1:5 (House of Commons Hansard, Storthes Hall Hospital, 2 Nov 1961). According to the hospital's management, part of the problem in attracting staff was its distance from the town centre and this led to questions being asked by local MPs in the House of Commons (UK parliament) (Reports and Statistical Tables, Storthes Hall Hospital 1949). Even the introduction of a subsidised bus service could not always compete with the other job opportunities in the town's chemical, textile and motor industries, which were much more accessible, had better working conditions and were equally, if not more generously, well-paid (House of Commons Hansard, Storthes Hall Hospital, 26 July 1955).

Just as the institution was not necessarily a "local" institution for its patients, neither was it always one for its staff. At the end of the 1940s, 19 European Voluntary Workers (EVWs) drawn from the refugee camps of Europe supplemented the employment of untrained nursing assistants as the hospital management sought to address the parlous staffing situation (Storthes Hall Management Group, 31 Dec 1949). This included specific recruitment drives at the hospital and campaigns in nearby towns but, as the years progressed, their reach extended, and the diversity of staff increased. From the mid-1950s, and as part of a general trend in the UK, hospital managers looked first to Ireland and then further afield.

By 1971, 24% of the nursing staff at Storthes Hall had been born outside of the UK (House of Commons Hansard, Huddersfield Hospitals, 11 Feb 1971). Significant numbers had come from Ireland (31), but many had travelled from Commonwealth territories and countries, including the West Indies (39), Mauritius (27), and Ghana (10) and they often faced outright hostility (McCrae and Nolan 2016, 220). Just as trade unions had lobbied for restriction on the employment of EVWs so too did they oppose the arrival of 29 new nurses who hailed from Nigeria and Jamaica, leading, once again, to questions being raised in parliament (Wrench 2000, 133–4; McCrae and Nolan 2016, 220). Local MPs and a spokesperson for the Ministry of Health clashed over whether the hostility rested with a "colour bar" (Yorkshire Post, 25 Nov 1955; Leeds Intelligencer 28 Nov 1955; House of Commons Hansard, Mental Hospital, Huddersfield, 14 Dec 1955) and this was not the only controversy that Storthes Hall would face. In 1967, *Sans Everything: A Case to Answer* was published by a psychotherapist,

Barbara Robb and the Aid for the Elderly in Government Institutions (AEGIS) group. Along with claims made about seven other hospitals, Storthes Hall became mired in a scandal relating to the mistreatment of geriatric patients and this was followed by lurid headlines in the press that spoke of "sex orgies" on hospital wards and of vulnerable patients being prescribed the contraceptive pill (Daily Mirror, 1 June 1965; Hide 2018, 741).

3 Oral History, Memory and the Narratives of Mental Health Care

The narrative of the hospital's complex and difficult development, which was beset by structural, logistical and funding issues can be contrasted with Anne Littlewood's *Storthes Hall Remembered* which was published in 2003. Littlewood, a former senior member of the nursing staff at the hospital, recognised that most of the memories she recorded were of "happy busy times" (Littlewood 2003, 5) but she was aware that they may have offered a "rose tinted" view and that patients who had spent time in the institution may have had a more "realistic view of the past" (Littlewood 2003, 5). Despite this potential dissonance, there were some notable absences in her book, and in the sample of interviews from the PHOA that have been used here. In the latter, for example, there was limited mentions of the arrival or place of foreign nurses in the patient accounts, while one staff member described a group of nurses recruited from Portugal as "hard-working" (Hisgett, Peter n.d.). Equally, there was very little said by staff or patients about the specifics of *Sans Everything* and to understand this, there has to be an understanding of the origins of the PHOA.

Speaking with David Storr, the Hospital Adminstrator who initiated the project, reveals that it was primarily a response to the imminent closure of Storthes Hall. Storr had previously worked at Fulbourne Hospital in Cambridge and had his own views about the changes that were taking place. He felt that community care was the right approach but it needed "a lot of resources" to be done in a "sympathetic and innovative way. Evidence was emerging [...] that the way in which resettlement was being tackled was not doing anybody any favours." Moreover, in Huddersfield at the time the project was conducted and as the hospital closure approached, concerns were building in relation to where patients would go and what would happen to the aging population from the psycho-geriatric wards. There were also concerns about drug and alcohol misuse, and those who "were still going to need a locked ward" (Storr 2020).

Storr was a member of the project steering group, which included other members of staff from the hospital and representatives from Pennine Heritage, a local history organisation based in nearby Hebden Bridge. Their aim was to "enable people who had worked, lived or had contact with the hospital to speak about their experiences, given that the Hospital was scheduled for closure [...] and to give a voice to some people whose recollections might not otherwise have been heard" (Storr 2020). The project was advertised to patients and staff in newsletters, and staff and patient meetings.

The interviews were conducted by volunteers who were recruited and trained by Pennine Heritage and, before the project began, they were given a tour of the hospital and briefed on how it functioned by hospital staff. As Storr remembered, little information was passed on relating to the history of the hospital and issues such as the accusations of patient mistreatment or discrimination against overseas staff were not included in the briefing. Those asking the questions were advised to begin by asking basic questions, such as what the interviewee's job was, if they were staff, or what ward they were on, if patients, and then to conduct relatively unstructured interviews that asked people to reflect on "what mattered to them about the hospital, the big moments, the contact." (Storr 2020).

At the end of the interviews, all participants were asked to sign what were described as Project Clearance Notes, which enabled them to agree to, or limit the use of their testimonies in future work. (Pennine Heritage, c.1986). These were very detailed, and tick boxes allowed signatories to opt out of having material from their interviews re-produced in a range of formats that included, museum, schools, television and radio broadcasts, and publications. A later iteration of the consent form removed the options and asked participants to specify their own restrictions, presumably because a significant minority of those taking part were ticking some of the boxes and limiting the reach of the project. Other patients and staff were happy for their work to be used, on the condition that their contribution was anonymised and in those cases their names have been redacted.

Despite the concerns about closure highlighted by Storr, both patients and staff spoke more generally about "control". Patients remembered locked doors and restrictions on movement. Name Redacted A explained if patients needed the toilet the nurse would say "you can't go to the toilet until I open the door [...] you couldn't just go the toilet everything were locked, I'm not kidding you!" (Name Redacted A, 1988) Staff too commented on the repressive nature of locked doors and Mrs Dibb, an accounts clerk who started work in 1940, recalled "you felt as if you had been trapped in prison" (Dibb, Mrs E J 1986).

As well as restricting the movement of patients, discipline in the hospital was also exercised through violence. According to former patient, Name Redacted B, there existed "what we called in those days the staff squad [...] I seen it in action and it bloody terrified me." The "staff squad" was seemingly called to deal with violent patients and "it was purely a physical assault [...] it did the job [...] the guy who caused it was made to know he had caused it". (Name Redacted B, 1988). By contrast, very few staff members talked about violence in the hospital and these silences remind us that, as Luisa Passerini (1983, 196) argues, there is no "work of memory" without a corresponding "work of forgetting". Passerini has shown how forgetting can be a way interviewees supress or distance themselves from difficult or traumatic experiences whereas, Freund has argued that silences can reflect a conscious form of agency and control. (Freund 2013)

Where it was remembered, the use of force was explained as a necessity. Mrs Kendall, who came to work in the occupational therapy department as it was being set up in 1953, and eventually became its head, explained that on some wards there were "epileptic patients who were very violent" and, on others, "young psychopaths who fought among themselves." For her, forcible restraint was needed to combat "the difficulties that the nurses had to deal with" (Kendall, Mr & Mrs 1986).

These examples of remembering and forgetting shine a light on the complexity inherent in the re-creation of historical narratives. Violence to patients sits at the nexus between Littlewood's "rose-tinted" account and that of the social historians and others who have sought to delve behind the vested interests of those conveying a "favourable image of institutions" (McCrae and Nolan 2016, XI). The shadow of Michel Foucault looms large here, and the recognition that patient identities are often recreated by sources which privilege medical power (Foucault 2003). Oral histories generally and the PHOA specifically in this case, appear to offer one way to resolve this imbalance but not all those taking part consented to having their memories used across the board. A very small amount of evidence that might have been used in this chapter had to be discounted on ethical grounds when the Project Clearance Notes were discovered by accident during an unrelated archival visit. Even when documented, the 'patients perspective' may not always be available to historians and for a larger, more detailed analysis of resources such as these, this may prove to be problematic.

Moreover, to some the use of personal memory as a source also remains problematic (Abrams 2016; Green 2004; Kansteiner 2002). Maurice Halbwachs and others have questioned how far "the wider social and cultural context in which remembering takes place" influences the way memories are constructed (Halbwachs 1992; Green 2004, 35). One of the first sociologists to study memory, Halbwachs emphasised that individual memories are shaped by dominant "social frameworks" through which group identities are formed (Halbwachs

1992). Indeed, although opportunities for patient stories to be told and heard have increased in recent years through developments such as group therapy, ward meetings and even survivor stories, these narratives are often situated within the boundaries of individual illness and their treatment regimes (Swartz 1996).

Yet some oral historians, historians of medicine, survivors, and those working within the field of Mad Studies have attempted to work outside of this framework (Green 2004; Davies 2001; Portelli 2020). Green, for example, argues "contemporary theorising around collective memory has paid too little attention to the capacity of individuals to reflect critically on both their own experience and practice and those of others." (Green 2010, 108). Portelli, on the other hand, highlights the "dialogical relationship" between the historian and the narrator and the "fluid, interactive and often more ambivalent dialogue" which allows space for personal experience to be recalled in ways that can challenge or subvert accepted narratives (Portelli 2020; Green 2004, 41). Indeed, as Thompson has highlighted, the capacity of oral histories to contest narratives that reflect dominant "social frameworks" and create independent accounts of the past has been shown by work carried out with marginalised and disempowered groups. (Thompson 2007, 57–58; Ellis, Kendal, and Taylor 2021).

As has already been shown, the interviews in the PHOA were framed by questions relating to Storthes Hall's place within a "dominant social framework" that involved the social and spatial separation of vulnerable individuals. However, the archive's strength was and is in the will of those who collected the testimonies to understand the hospital's history, good and bad, by documenting the experiences of people who worked and lived there. The relatively semi-structured approach to the interviews consisted of open questions based around general themes such as first impressions of the hospital and relationships between staff and patients. On reading the full transcripts of the interviews it is clear this achieved its aim and allowed space for interviewees to explore issues and experiences that were most important to them at the time. Clearly the timing of the interviews was also important, and the planned closure of the hospital offered both patients and staff a chance to reflect on life at the hospital and what might be lost.

4   First Impressions and Longer-Term Perceptions

Understandably, the issue of separation and the stigma that were apparent in official reports were also prominent in the patients' first impressions of Storthes Hall. Name Redacted A, who was first admitted in 1947, for example, offered a poignant account of his first impressions of Storthes Hall, remembering "I'd heard a lot about this place before I came here you know, I knew what it [was]. I never thought I'd end up here" (Name Redacted A, 1988). Name Redacted B recalled the hospital was "very much cut off from the world" and that he was "a bit fearsome" before lamenting how, at the time, he hoped "Storthes Hall was a stop in a life" but it became "a long stop for 25 years" (Name Redacted B, 1988). Eric S, on the other hand, remembered having no negative perceptions of the hospital commenting simply that "it looked to be alright for me". But this was unusual and may have been because Eric "knew a few patients" and his familiarity with people in the hospital may have reduced the sense of stigma surrounding it (S, Eric 1986).

Frank Holroyde began work as an untrained attendant at the hospital in 1926. He remembered being "frightened out of my wits [...] [be]cause it was a strange world" (Holroyde 1986) and 50 years later Mr Carrisites, who worked in the upholstery department in the 1980s, remembered thinking he would "see strange things and hear strange things, and meet strange people" (Carrisites, Mr n.d.). By contrast, W. E. Thompson, a member of the psychiatric medical staff, saw his appointment in the 1930s as "very exciting really, because, psychiatry in those days was an 'in' thing [and] I was very impressed with the general aura of the place" (Thompson 1986). Jackie Reed, a nurse who began work at Storthes Hall in 1979, and eventually became Deputy Director of Nursing, remembered similarly positive first impressions. She found "when you actually got inside I thought that the facilities here are excellent" and the patients "well looked after". Even here then, the community understanding of mental hospitals was pervasive and she noted that the conditions inside the hospital were better than expected, commenting it was an "old hospital and the reputation that any hospitals have [...] you judge from the outside" (Reed n.d.).

Such findings reflect similar points made by Geoffrey Reaume about the importance of families and communities, and the place of prejudice and misunderstanding in their responses to mental illness (Reaume 2009). While research has shown that local communities could be both understanding and tolerant, as well as intolerant of both the patients and treatment facilities on their doorstep (Ellis 2013), the participants in this case had the advantage of seeing things for themselves and there was a contrast to be found in their longer-term experiences of hospital life. Despite the fearsome reputation of some members of staff, Name Redacted A remembered others who were friendly towards him, (Name Redacted A, 1988) while Vera Clegg who worked as kitchen maid at the hospital and was "a bit frightened at first" found she got "very attached" to the patients as "you felt they needed someone for a little bit of friendliness." (Clegg 1986). Similarly, Nancy B was admitted to Storthes

Hall after suffering a violent breakdown in 1958. Initially, she spent a month in confinement in a padded cell and was then moved to one of the hospital's geriatric wards. After vividly remembering the distress of her breakdown and confinement, she painted a far more tranquil picture of her time on the ward, describing the nurses who cared for her as, "lovely", and the hospital as, "a beautiful place". She also remembered the companionship provided by a ward cat "They called it Mick, I called it Micky [...] it used to come and sleep on my bed" (B, Nancy 1987).

Some staff and patients spoke of changes within the hospital from the 1950s and 60s, which appeared to present the regime as more relaxed and reflected the reformist "Therapeutic Community" approach highlighted by Fussinger (2011) which aimed to "humanize" psychiatric institutions. According to Mrs Kendall, the introduction of tranquilising drugs in the 1950s significantly reduced violence amongst the patients and improved their quality of life (Littlewood 2003, 120–121). When staff "hadn't the drugs", she stated, "they were just custodians [...] and everything was locked, windows, everything was locked" (Kendall, Mr & Mrs 1986). By the end of the 1960s some patients were allowed to go out unaccompanied and even visit local bars. Name Redacted A. explained how he could "go to town in the morning shopping" and "go out on a Saturday drinking and gambling". (Name Redacted A, 1988). As Gittins noted, aspects of life and treatment at Severalls changed significantly, even if to outsiders it did not appear to (Gittins, 3) and Littlewood writes of social activities, such as dances, concerts, day trips and sporting activities and even, from 1974, a hospital pub, the Toby Jug (Littlewood 2003, 66–78).

The examples here foreshadow more recent scholarship which has highlighted the loss of friendships (Gittins 1998, 57, 153; Calabria et al. 2021) and the loss of the relatively safe institutional spaces (Taylor 2015, 269) that resulted from the closure programme. Significantly too, the emphasis on a narrative of progress, of a turning point, becomes complicated by a longer-term story of community engagement. Even in the nineteenth and early twentieth centuries, some asylum patients spent time on excursions or took part in other activities, such as walking parties that were claimed to be both diverting and therapeutic (Ellis 2013). At Storthes Hall, some patients were taken on extra-institutional holidays in the 1930s (Littlewood 2003, 74–76) and, in one year in the 1940s, "motor tours" took patients to a wide variety of venues including the theatre, pantomimes, the circus, flower shows, agricultural shows and even to the centre of Huddersfield to see the future Queen, Her Royal Highness Princess Elizabeth, visit the town with her husband (Storthes Hall Management Group Hospital Management Committee 1948).

With a wide range of activities in the hospital grounds, including presentations by invited guests, and even free admission for patients at the local football (Huddersfield Town) and rugby league clubs, (Reports and Statistical Tables Relating to Storthes Hall Hospital 1948) we can see a longer-term story of community interaction that clouds both the perception of change and of distance from wider society, even if not all patients were able to share, or were even allowed the same opportunities.

5   Hospital Closure and Community Care

Despite these activities, the sense of distance and of social and spatial separation became a defining feature of the discussions around closure. Letters to local newspapers revealed questions raised by church groups, local councillors, mental health charities and local residents, as well as the relatives of patients affected by the closure of Storthes Hall (Haigh 5 June 1987, *Huddersfield District Newspapers*; Heathcote 5 May 1984, *Huddersfield Examiner*; 29 Jan 1988, *Huddersfield Examiner*). The focus of these articles and letters included the impact that the loss of in-patient services would have on the individuals being moved into the community. In one letter, the daughter of a patient questioned the hospital's closure because the decision had been made "without any thought at all as to how people's lives will be affected" and this was clearly on the minds of those interviewed by the Pennine Heritage team (Haigh 5 June 1987, *Huddersfield District Newspapers*). Name Redacted B spoke of his concerns, saying "what happens out there I don't know, I don't think about it to be honest, I'm frightened to think about it." (Name Redacted B, 1988). Without the appropriate level of support, he feared he might slip back into the alcoholism that had led to his admission to Storthes Hall, seventeen years earlier but he wondered what level of support would be there for him. "I've got a son", he said, "and I wouldn't deploy myself on him and his family [...] there is no obvious care and concern shown [in the community] [...] I've had it done to me [before] they've turned and walked away, it doesn't give you confidence." For him, Storthes Hall was that safe space and he explained, "I don't look upon this place as a hospital at all anymore, it's my home [...] where all my friendships are [...] my mates, my way of life's here." (Name Redacted B, 1988). Name Redacted A's thoughts on his imminent move into the community reflect a more nuanced narrative. He commented "you don't want to be tied up in a place like this when you're young same as I was." But now approaching his seventieth birthday he reflected on being able to live a lifestyle in the hospital which involved having a radio, reading the newspaper, going out of the hospital shopping and visiting the public house on Saturdays, before concluding "I enjoy it here [...] I'm happy, it's all I want." (Name Redacted A, 1988).

Both Name Redacted B's and Name Redacted A's caution at their discharge mirrored the apprehension of their first arrival at Storthes Hall and of the unknown. Similar unease over the move to community care could be seen in the views of some staff members. Mrs Kendall, the occupational therapist, for example, expressed concerns about the contradictory nature of attitudes towards patients in the community. When discussing the opening up of the hospital she commented:

> The public at this stage I think were a lot to blame because while they wanted the doors open, if any of the patients went down into the village and did things that were considered anti-social or they thought they were dangerous, there was a very big hue and cry [...] the public at large [was not] prepared to take on these people and still aren't. I mean you have just to go into a district and mention putting in a house, or opening something for patients [...] there is a hue and cry: "we cannot have these people living among us". So how far have we come? (Kendall, Mr & Mrs 1986)

The potential violence of patients also featured in the negotiations that Dr Tabarek Hossain, a consultant psychiatrist at St Luke's Hospital, had with a local church. As the president of Relative Concern, a then new mental health charity, it was hoped that they could hire the church, renovate it and have sessions on things such as cooking and handicrafts for discharged patients in the community. According to Hossain, the contact at the church asked if guards, bars on the windows and locks on the doors would be needed.

> I had no doubt in my own mind that he has got the mental picture of persons who are very unmanageable, who are rough, who are aggressive, who are violent, who do not know fire regulations and all that kind of thing, which is just utter nonsense. Anybody can walk through Storthes Hall and see the vast majority of patients are no different from us in the community. So this stigma lives on and we don't know how you can really, kind of, burst it. (Hossain, M. M. T. 1986)

In other cases, concerns were less about violence than they were about a reintroduction into the "real world". An article in the local press reported that long-term Storthes Hall patients who had "never seen modern traffic on a road before and were expecting to see horses and carts" would be a danger to themselves and to others. According to members of Kirkburton Road Safety

Committee, these fears had initially been raised by staff at Storthes Hall during a visit by representatives from the local Police to look at arrangements for rehabilitation cases ("Safety Fears" Circa mid-1980s, unreferenced article). The claims were countered by David Whalley, support services manager at Storthes Hall. He explained that the hospital "was not such a closed and confined community as many people thought [...] many patients come and go quite regularly and are well used to traffic conditions both locally and in the towns." Mr Whalley also commented "road safety is taught as part of the rehabilitation process, and patients are taken off into town centres with staff as part of the training." ("Safety Fears" circa mid-1980s, unreferenced article).

Representatives from some churches in Huddersfield and hospital staff took more positive action, establishing a volunteer run "friendship centre" for former patients. The initiative was welcomed by Eddie Jefferson, the general manager of Storthes Hall, at a meeting organised by the Community and Mental Health unit of Huddersfield Health Authority to discuss fears about patients from Storthes Hall being "dispersed" into the community. Mr Jefferson stated volunteers had always played an important role in the hospital but "the need for this while the Hospital is closing is greater than ever" and "members of the community" could play "a great part in helping and supporting discharged patients to make a new life." ("Concern over Hall patients" 5 June 1987, *Huddersfield District Newspapers*).

6   Conclusion

There can be little doubt that Douglas Spencer's desire to preserve the histories of hospitals like Storthes Hall, reflected their ubiquitous nature in the landscape of care and treatment. It was, however, their impending closure that explains the narratives recorded in the PHOA. As a starting point, official reports and documents show just how complex Storthes Hall's history and development was. The parlous nature of staff:patient ratios, issues around recruitment, the hostility faced by some overseas staff, and the scandalous treatment of some patients, only seem to confirm some of the very worst representations of mental hospitals in the twentieth century. The PHOA offers a rare opportunity to add to the piecemeal nature of the "official" historical record but the relative silences on some of these issues reveals both its strength and its weaknesses. On the one hand, the apparently open nature of both the questions, and the willingness of the interviewers to let the patients and staff talk about the issues that were important to them, appears to emphasise the lack of an agenda in the process of capturing memories. On the other, Storr's recollections of the

PHOA project's origins and his own views about the processes of deinstitution-alisation and its limitations show that some of the outcomes may have been pre-determined.

As a result, we are left with a somewhat positive and progressive narrative of the hospital, where things only improved and barriers with the community were only broken down – what Littlewood recognised as a potentially "rose-tinted" view. This, however, has to be framed in how both patients and staff saw the prospects for deinstitutionalisation and what parts the local community might play in that. The apparent openness of the questions belied the context of closure and the sense of loss and foreboding that emanated from them. Fears about what faced patients in the real world can be contrasted, somewhat ironi-cally, with the trepidation that many faced when encountering Storthes Hall for the first time and there are two things to consider here. The first of these is the patients themselves. We can be sure that not all patients, or staff for that matter, became as settled as the ones that are included here. In addition, not all patients were able to engage in all of Storthes Hall's activities either within the hospital grounds, or as part of the wider community. A different cohort may have spoken more clearly to the darker side of its history and presented a very different narrative to the prospect of deinstitutionalisation. As historians, for example, we would have liked to have known more about the impact of low levels of staffing, of overcrowding, of the colour bar, and of the scandals on the patient experience but these are all sadly lacking.

The second issue was the pervasiveness of how some members of the local community viewed Storthes Hall and that includes people who had either lived or worked there. In this respect we have to recognise that patients came from those communities and this shaped both how they viewed the prospects for their admission and also their discharge. The battle that Spencer, and his colleagues and predecessors faced, was to overcome that othering of mental health hospitals and, more importantly, the people within them. As we have seen, what we might call folk- knowledge of institutions followed people into Storthes Hall and it followed them out again. This was despite the attempts at community interaction, of which the PHOA was just one example, and despite the more recent research which has sought to question how far local communi-ties lobbied against asylums and mental hospitals in their local area (Reinarz, Mooney 2009; Ellis 2013).

Acknowledgements

The authors are grateful to Dr Verusca Calabria for her suggestions on an initial draft of this chapter and to the volume's reviewers for their comments. Thanks are also due to Adele Owens and Lauren Le Ber for some of the detail on the early discussions relating to the Storthes Hall site.

References

Aaslestad, Petter. 2019. *The Patient as Text: The Role of the Narrator in Psychiatric Notes, 1890–1990*. Abingdon: Radliffe.

Abrams, Lynn. 2016. *Oral History Theory*. London: Routledge.

Name Redacted A. Storthes Hall Oral History Recordings. 1986–1988. University of Huddersfield. Heritage Quay Archive Collection. SH/4/ Patient Group 3, 7 Jan 1988.

B., Nancy. 1987. Storthes Hall Oral History Recordings. 1986–1988. University of Huddersfield. Heritage Quay Archive Collection. SH/4/Patient Group 3.

Name Redacted B. 1988. Storthes Hall Oral History Recordings. 1986–1988. University of Huddersfield. Heritage Quay Archive Collection. SH/4/Patient Group 2.

Bartlett, Peter, and Ralph Sandland. 2007. *Mental Health Law, Policy and Practice*. Oxford: Oxford University Press.

Beckman, Emily, Elizabeth Nelson, and Modupe Labode. 2022. "Voices from the Newspaper Club: Patient Life at a State Psychiatric Hospital (1988–1992)." *Journal of Medical Humanities* 43 (1): 179–195.

Bornat, Joanna. 2005. "Recycling the Evidence: Different Approaches to the Reanalysis of Gerontological Data." *Forum Qualitative Sozialforschung / Forum: Qualitative Social Research* 6 (1), Art. 42, http://nbn-resolving.de/urn:nbn:de:0114-fqs0501424 (accessed June 4, 2021).

Brumby, Alice. 2015. "'A Painful and Disagreeable Position': Rediscovering Patient Narratives and Evaluating the Difference between Policy and Experience for institutionalized Veterans with Mental Disabilities, 1924–1931." *First World War Studies*. 6; no 1: 37–55.

Calabria, Verusca. 2019. "Insider Stories from the Asylum: Peer and Staff-Patient relationships". In *Narrating Illness: Prospects and Constraints*, edited by Joanna Davidson and Yomna Saber, 1–12. Oxford: Inter-Disciplinary Press.

Calabria, Verusca, Di Bailey and Graham Bowpitt. 2021. "More than Bricks and Mortar: Meaningful Care Practices in the Old State Mental Hospitals". In *Voices in the History of Madness: Patient and Practitioner Perspectives*, edited by Rob Ellis, Sarah Kendall, and Steven J. Taylor, 191–215. Cham: Palgrave Macmillan.

Carrisites, Mr. n.d. *Storthes Hall Oral History Recordings*. 1986–1988. University of Huddersfield. Heritage Quay Archive Collection. SH/4/Not Listed group 2, 5 tapes.

Chaney, Sarah, and Jennifer Walke. 2019. "Mansions in the Orchard: Architecture, Asylum and Community in Twentieth-Century Mental Health Care". In *Communicating the History of Medicine: Perspectives on Audiences and Impact*, edited by

Solveig Jülich and Sven Widmalm. Manchester: Manchester University Press (accessed August 18, 2020).

Clegg, Vera. 1986. *Storthes Hall Oral History Recordings*. 1986–1988. University of Huddersfield. Heritage Quay Archive Collection. SH/4/Vera C (A and B sides).

Coleborne, Catherine. 2020. *Why talk about Madness. Bringing History into the Conversation*. Cham: Palgrave Macmillan.

Coleborne, Catherine, and Dolly MacKinnon. 2011. *Exhibiting Madness in Museums. Remembering Psychiatry through Collections and Display*. Abingdon: Routledge.

Crang, Mike. 1998. *Cultural Geography*. London: Routledge.

Craze, Alison. 2014. *Asylum to Community Care: A History of Brookwood Hospital Told by Those who Worked and Lived There*. Publisher not identified.

Crossley, Nick. 2006. *Contesting Psychiatry: Social Movements in Mental Health*. London: Routledge.

N.A. "Mental Patients Given the Pill." *Daily Mirror,* 1 June 1965, 7.

Davies, Kerry. 2001. "'Silent and Censured Travellers'? Patients' Narratives and Patients' Voices: Perspectives on the History of Mental Illness Since 1948:" *Social History of Medicine* 14, no. 2: 267–292.

Dibb, Mrs E. J. 1986. *Storthes Hall Oral History Recordings*. 1986–1988. University of Huddersfield. Heritage Quay Archive Collection. SH/4/Unbundled Tapes 1–10.

Ellis, Rob. 2013. "'A Constant Irritation to the Townspeople'? Local, Regional and National Politics and London's County Asylums at Epsom", *Social History of Medicine* 26, no.4: 653–671.

Ellis, Rob. 2015. "Without Decontextualisation: the Stanley Royd Museum and the Progressive History of Mental Health Care." *History of Psychiatry* 26, no.3: 332–347.

Ellis, Rob. 2020. *London and its Asylums, 1888–1914. Politics and Madness*. London: Palgrave Macmillan.

Ellis, Rob, Sarah Kendal, and Steven J. Taylor. 2021. *Voices in the History of Madness. Personal and Professional Perspective on Mental Health and Illness*. London: Palgrave Macmillan.

Fifty-ninth Report of the Commissioners in Lunacy. 1905. https://parlipapers.proquest.com/parlipapers (accessed March 21, 2020).

Foucault, Michel. 2003. *The Birth of the Clinic: An Archaeology of Medical Perception*. Routledge Classics. Taylor & Francis.

Freund, Alexander. 2013. "Toward an Ethics of Silence? Negotiating Off-the-Record Events and Identity in Oral History." In *Oral History Off the Record: Toward an Ethnography of Practice*, edited by Anna Sheftel and Stacey Zembrzyck, 223–238. New York: Palgrave.

Fussinger, Catherine. 2011. "'Therapeutic Community', Psychiatry's Reformers and Antipsychiatrists: Reconsidering Changes in the Field of Psychiatry after World War II." *History of Psychiatry* 22:2: 146–163.

Gallagher, Mark. 2018. "From Associations to Action: Mental Health and Patient Politics of Subsidiarity in Scotland." *Palgrave Communication* 4, no. 34: 1–11.

Gittins, Diana. 1998. *Madness in its Place: Narratives of Severalls Hospital 1913–1997*. London, New York: Routledge.

Glenside Hospital Museum. n.d. Psychiatric Hospitals 1861–1994, *Mental Health Treatment from the 1850s to the 1990s*. http://www.glensidemuseum.org.uk/psychiatric-hospital-1861–1994/ (accessed August 18, 2020).

Green, Anna. 2004. "Individual Remembering and Collective Memory". *Oral History Journal* 32, no 2. 35–44.

Green, Anna. 2010. "Can Memory be Collective?". In *The Oxford Handbook of Oral History*, edited by Donald A. Ritchie, 96–111. Oxford: Oxford University Press.

Haigh, Jean. Letter to *Huddersfield District Newspapers* 5 June 1987.

Halbwachs, Maurice. 1992. *On Collective Memory*. Chicago: University of Chicago Press.

Heathcote, E. Letter to *Huddersfield Examiner*, 5 May 1984.

Hide, Louise. 2018, "In Plain Sight: Open Doors, Mixed Sex Wards and Sexual Abuse in English Psychiatric Hospitals, 1950s to Early 1990s." *Social History of Medicine* 31, no. 4: 732–753.

Hisgett, Peter. N.d. *Storthes Hall Oral History Recordings*. 1986–1988. University of Huddersfield. Heritage Quay Archive Collection. SH/4/Unbundled Tapes 31–40.

Holroyde, Frank. 1986. *Storthes Hall Oral History Recordings*. 1986–1988. University of Huddersfield. Heritage Quay Archive Collection. SH/4/Not Listed group 1.

Hossain, Tabarek. 1986. *Storthes Hall Oral History Recordings*. 1986–1988. University of Huddersfield. Heritage Quay Archive Collection. SH/4/ Unbundled Tapes 11–20 Not listed Group 2.

House of Commons Hansard. 1955. Mental Hospital, Huddersfield. 4 Dec 1955. https://api.parliament.uk/historic-hansard/commons/1955/dec/14/mental-hospital-huddersfield (accessed August 18, 2020).

House of Commons Hansard. 1955. Staff Recruitment. Storthes Hall Hospital, 26 July 1955. https://hansard.parliament.uk/commons/1955-07-26/debates/55623f4e-19de-41ae-9162-,8f3b82f7822b/StaffRecruitmentStorthesHallHospital (accessed June 23, 2020).

House of Commons Hansard. 1961. Storthes Hall Hospital (Staff Transport). 2 Nov 1961. https://hansard.parliament.uk/Commons/1961-11-02/debates/3b9eaa69-c7ac-4c28-aac3-218187bffad1/StorthesHallHospital(StaffTransport) (accessed August 18, 2020).

House of Commons Hansard. 1971. Huddersfield Hospitals (Nurses), 11 Feb 1971. https://hansard.parliament.uk/Commons/1971-02-11/debates/803c6f21-084b-49c3-a5fb-903dceed5b17/HuddersfieldHospitals(Nurses) (accessed August 18, 2020).

Huddersfield District Newspapers, 5 June 1987. "Concern over Hall patients".

Huddersfield Examiner 29 Jan 1988.

Kansteiner, Wulf. 2002. "Finding Meaning in Memory: A Methodological Critique of Collective Memory Studies." *History and Theory* 41. no 2. 179–197.

Kendall, Mr & Mrs. 1986. *Storthes Hall Oral History Recordings. 1986–1988*. University of Huddersfield. Heritage Quay Archive Collection. SH/4/ Unbundled Tapes, 11–20.

Leeds Intelligencer 28 Nov 1955.

Littlewood, Ann. 2003. *Storthes Hall Remembered*. Huddersfield: University of Huddersfield.

M., Harold. 1988. *Storthes Hall Oral History Recordings*. 1986–1988. University of Huddersfield. Heritage Quay Archive Collection. SH/4/Patient Group 2.

McCrae, Niall, and Peter Nolan. 2016. *The Story of Nursing in British Mental Hospitals: Echoes from the Corridors*. Taylor & Francis Group.

Memories of St David's Hospital, Carmarthen, Wales. Heritage Lottery Fund Project. 2016. http://stdavidshospital.co.uk/ (accessed August 18, 2020).

Michigan Radio: Michigan's NPR News Leader, *Oral history project documents life at Traverse City mental hospital*. https://www.michiganradio.org/post/oral-history-project-documents-life-traverse-city-mental-hospital (accessed August 18, 2020).

Parr, Hester, Chris Philo, and Nicola Burns. 2003. "'That Awful Place was Home': Reflections on the Contested Meanings of Craig Dunain Asylum." *Scottish Geographical Journal* 119. no.4: 341–360.

Passerini , Luisa. 1983. "Memory". *History Workshop Journal* 15: 195–196.

Payne, Sarah. 1999. "Outside the Walls of the Asylum? Psychiatric Treatment in the 1980s and the 1990s". In *Outside the Walls of the Asylum*, edited by Peter Bartlett and David Wright, 244–65. London and New Brunswick: The Athlone Press.

Pennine Heritage, c.1986, Storthes Hall Accession Details, Clearance Notes.

Portelli, Alessandro. "A Dialogical Relationship. An Approach to Oral History." https://pdfslide.net/documents/a-dialogical-relationship-an-approach-to-oral-history.html (accessed August 18, 2020).

Porter, Roy. 1985. "The Patients' View. Doing Medical History from Below." *Theory and Society* 14:2: 175–198.

Raferty, James. 1996. "The Decline of Asylum or the Poverty of the Concept". In *Asylum in the Community*; edited by Dylan Tomlinson and John Carrier, 18–30. London: Routledge.

Reaume, Geoffrey. 2009. *Remembrance of Patients Past: Patient Life at the Toronto Hospital for the Insane, 1870–1940*. Toronto: University of Toronto Press.

Reed, Miss Jackie. N.d. *Storthes Hall Oral History Recordings*. 1986–1988. University of Huddersfield. Heritage Quay Archive Collection. SH/4/Unbundled Tapes 51–60 and 61–70.

Reinarz, Johnathan, and Graham Mooney, eds. 2009. *Permeable Walls. Historical Perspectives on Hospital and Asylum Visiting*. Amsterdam: Rodopi.

S., Eric. 1986. *Storthes Hall Oral History Recordings. 1986–1988.* University of Huddersfield. Heritage Quay Archive Collection. SH/4/Patient Group 1.

Spencer, Douglas A. 1985. "Some Historical Records on the Mansion Hospital and Storthes Hall Hospital, Kirkburton, Huddersfield." West Yorkshire: Unpublished Manuscript.

Storthes Hall Group Hospital Management Committee No. 12. 1948. Leeds Regional Hospital Board. Reports and Statistical Tables Relating to Storthes hall Hospital. Kirkburton. https://wellcomecollection.org/ (accessed August 18, 2020).

Storthes Hall Group Hospital Management Committee. No. 12. 1949. Leeds Regional Hospital Board. Reports and Statistical Tables Relating to Storthes hall Hospital, Kirkburton. https://wellcomecollection.org/ (accessed August 18, 2020).

Storthes Hall Oral History Recordings. 1986–1988. University of Huddersfield. Heritage Quay Archive Collection. STH/6/4.

Storr, David. 2020. Oral history interview conducted by R. Light at Pennine Heritage, Hebden Bridge. Ellis/Light Collection.

Swartz, Sally. 1996. "Shrinking: A Postmodern Perspective on Psychiatric Case Histories". *South African Journal of Psychiatry* 26.150–156.

Taylor, Barbara. 2015. *The Last Asylum. A Memoir of Madness in Our Times,* Chicago: University of Chicago Press.

Testimony: Inside Stories of Mental Health Care! https://www.webarchive.org.uk/way back/archive/20121013223331/http://www.insidestories.org/ (accessed June 18, 2020).

Thompson, W. E. 1986. Storthes Hall Oral History Recordings. 1986–1988. University of Huddersfield. Heritage Quay Archive Collection. SH/4/Not listed Group 2.

Thomson, Alistair. 2007. "Four Paradigm Transformations in Oral History." *The Oral History Review* 34:1. 49–70.

Thurgood, Graham J. 2002. "Nurses and Nursing in Huddersfield: 1870–1960". In *Aspects of Huddersfield: Discovering Local History,* 111–126. Barnsley: Wharncliffe Books.

Thurgood, Graham J. 2008. *A History of Nursing in Halifax and Huddersfield 1870–1960.* Unpublished doctoral thesis, University of Huddersfield.

Thurgood, Graham J. 2010. "Nurses' Voices from the Archives". *Journal of the Society of Archivists.* 31, no. 2: 135–147.

Turner, John, Rhodri Hayward, Katherine Angel, et al. 2015. "The History of Mental Health Services in Modern England: Practitioner Memories and the Direction of Future Research." *Medical History,* 59, no. 4: 599–624.

University of Exeter, Centre for Medical History. 2019. *Remembering the Mental Hospital.* https://humanities.exeter.ac.uk/history/research/centres/ medicalhistory/past /rememberingthementalhospital/ (accessed August 18, 2020).

Unreferenced Newspaper Cuttings. Circa mid 1980s. "Safety Fears". Folder 6. *Yorkshire Post,* 25 Nov 1955.

West Yorkshire Archive Service. C416/1/275 Storthes Hall Asylum Minute book, Vol 2: Apr 1904-Mar 1906, 9 Nov 1905.

West Yorkshire Archive Service. C416/1/275. Storthes Hall Asylum Minute book, Vol 1: Oct 1898-Feb 1904.

West Yorkshire Archive Service. WRC/3/15. Asylums Committee Minute Book 1897–1899.

Wrench, John, 2000. "British Unions and Racism: Organisational Dilemmas in an Unsympathetic Climate." In *Trade Unions, Immigration, and Immigrants in Europe, 1960–1993: A Comparative Study of the Attitudes and Actions of Trade Unions in Seven West European Countries*, edited by Rinus Penninx and Judith Roosblad, 133–156. New York: Berghahn Books.

CHAPTER 5

From Paternalism to Social Inclusion? User Organisations' Narratives of Psychiatric Services in Sweden

Veikko Pelto-Piri and Jenny Wetterling

Abstract

Service users of psychiatry and their organisations have for decades been trying to convey users' narratives on mental distress and its treatment. This work has made an impact; the trend is towards a humanistic psychiatric care and support; a journey from paternalism to social inclusion. Our aim in this chapter is to describe the user organisations' narratives of psychiatric services. The method for analysis is from narrative art history focusing on 1) transformation, 2) desire for and 3) lack of.

The user's organisations in Sweden started as a radical left-wing activist movement in the 1960s, supported by anti-psychiatry intellectuals. They managed to influence the public opinion and policy makers, which resulted in the deinstitutionalisation and humanisation of psychiatry. The following period was characterised by user organisations acting like trade unions moving towards a more dialogical work with the psychiatric services. Their major contribution was to influence the development of the new psychiatry based on outpatient care and community-based homes. Today the user organisations are more integrated in the psychiatric services and an active partner in co-creation and co-production of psychiatric services.

The user organisations, together with other stakeholders, have successfully contributed to a transformation of psychiatry. The large mental hospitals have closed; there has been an increased access to healthcare and to the quality of life for many of its service users. Still, there are difficulties, like the lack of support for the users who are most severely affected by mental distress, and different kinds of coercion. These problems need to be addressed at the policy level, rather than in the psychiatric health care system. To be successful there is a lot to learn from history where user organisations have acted as activists and tough trade union representatives. More than ever, free user organisations are needed that can give a voice to those who are unable to argue for their rights themselves. Then, maybe, we could move towards social inclusion; a society where we are "Leaving No One Behind".

Keywords

Coercion – narratives – policy – psychiatric services – serious mental illness – service users – values

1   The Conflicting Narratives of Psychiatry

In many cases, suffering from a serious mental illness is something that affects and significantly changes a person's life. Mental illness and disability affect our feelings and thoughts, which means that we often end up in a more vulnerable situation than otherwise. Maybe that's why many of us also feel afraid of the idea that mental illness can affect any of us. Many would like to see mental illness as something that affects others, even though at the same time we know that it is one of the most common forms of illness today. Knowledge about mental illness has increased rapidly in recent years, but there is still much left before we as a society and as fellow humans have a view of mental illness that is free from prejudice and ignorance. The unique individual with her experiences, needs and aspirations should be the obvious starting point for on how society's care and support is designed. (A reflection by Jenny Wetterling, a service user representative.)

For decades, service users of psychiatry and their organisations have been trying to convey users' narratives, as the one above, on mental distress and of the need for treatment and support. This work has made an impact. It is a development that can be characterised as a journey from paternalism to social inclusion, but this journey is not without obstacles. The history of psychiatry and the present provide examples of how the service user's perspective has been overruled by other stakeholders' theoretical considerations, personal beliefs and biomedical conditions.

Our aim in this chapter is to describe, firstly, some of the user organisations' narratives of psychiatric services in Sweden, secondly, how these narratives have been an answer to the psychiatric discourse, and, thirdly, how the service users influenced this discourse and the development of psychiatry. When we use the word discourse, we mean that professionals and policymakers have formed a discursive system for psychiatry. This is a system that leads to psychiatrization, creating a narrow framework for the interpretation of psychological distress and its treatment, which gives the psychiatric system control over the area of mental health (Logan and Karter 2022). The psychiatric discourse is formed in relation to medical ethics and has changed over time. The discourse strongly affects the communication opportunities for all stakeholders (Stacey 2016). Stakeholders that criticise the psychiatric services need to be understood in relation to the different perspectives of medical ethics in order to be taken seriously by other stakeholders in psychiatry. These normative perspectives of medical ethics are an important factor in the discursive system of psychiatry and are a part of psychiatry's immaterial heritage, as well as the users organisations' narratives. Therefore, the three perspectives of medical ethics will be presented and used in the analysis of narratives about change of the Swedish psychiatry. The method for analysis is from narrative art history focusing on 1) transformation, 2) desire for and 3) lack of (Kemp 1996). Such a structure fits in well with our aim since it gives us the questions that we find important.

1. What form of transformation has taken place in psychiatry over the last hundred years?
2. Which lack of, and desire for, was expressed in professionals' and policymakers' narratives in order to create the existing psychiatric services?
3. Which lack of, and desire for, did the users' and their organisations' narratives focus on when arguing for a change to the existing services?
4. What was the organisational narrative about the way of working as a user organisation?

We used these questions to understand the broad lines of the historical development of Swedish psychiatry and present a personal interpretation of this development as an essay, but first we will present the discussion on mental distress in Sweden and the ethical perspectives that have emerged over time.

Psychiatry is a value-laden activity where conflicting narratives have been competing about whose views should apply in psychiatric care and treatment. Often, different stakeholders cannot even agree on what causes psychiatric distress in the first place. Two well-known journalists and debaters in Sweden have given examples of various explanations of mental distress apparent in the Swedish context (Fredriksson and Moberg 2020). From the Middle Ages onwards, symptoms of mental distress could be interpreted as the work of the devil or as a punishment for sins committed. In the nineteenth century, physicians began to argue that mental distress is a condition that they should deal with. In Sweden, the mentally distressed were divided into two groups; the curable ones who were to be cared for in hospitals and the incurable ones who needed asylum. During the twentieth century, several models were developed to understand mental distress. The first to gain a strong position in Sweden was the psychodynamic perspective. The model was often used in Sweden to explain the cause of mental distress with early experiences of the individual. The biomedical model gradually replaced this perspective. The use of psychiatric medications has sharply increased and mental distress is commonly regarded as brain diseases caused by chemical imbalances that can be corrected with disease-specific drugs (Fredriksson and Moberg 2020). Many people, as the early user's movement, criticised this perspective. Instead, they emphasised that the causes of mental distress are to be found in injustice in society, such as stigmatization, coercion, and economic discrimination. These factors for mental distress can be best addressed by creating a society with social justice and respect for human rights (see Table 5.1; Pelto-Piri and Kjellin 2021; Fredriksson and Moberg 2020). This paradigm for mental health was advocated by the Social democratic movement in the last decades of the twentieth century (SOU 2006).

There is also a growing body of knowledge concerning the interaction between human cognitive functions, social function and symptoms of mental distress. An increasing number of neuropsychiatric examinations and the emergence of different psycho-pedagogical methods reflect this. Today, it is a common view, also among the user organisations, to explain mental distress as multifactorial and therefore treatment should be person-centred (NSPH 2018).

1.1　Values in Psychiatry

As mentioned, psychiatry is a value-laden activity, and it is possible to claim that psychiatry is more value-laden than other health-care specialities (Fulford 2007). There are several reasons for this claim.[1] One reason is that stakeholders do not agree on what causes psychiatric distress and what treatment is needed. Another reason is that a diagnosis is seldom based upon objective measurements; it is rather the assessment of the patient's and other people's narratives about the symptoms, life situations and functional disability (Fulford 2007; Sadler 2004). Different interpretations by different stakeholders can result in different opinions about treatment since psychiatry is focusing on areas of human life where concepts such as normality, identity, and value preferences are more central in the diagnosing process than in other specialties in healthcare (Thornton 2007). A third reason supporting this claim is that psychiatric services have the right to use coercive care and measures. So, staff members in mental health care often must manage conflicting values. Weighing different values in meetings with the patient becomes even more complicated since mental distress can affect the patient's autonomy and possibilities to communicate. Below, we are going to present three different normative ethical perspectives on how meetings with patients should be framed (Pelto-Piri,

---

1　This section is a shortened and updated version of "Normative Ethics in Staff Members' Encounters with Patients" by Pelto-Piri (2015, 13–18).

Engström, and Engström 2013; Pelto-Piri and Kjellin 2021), a framing having a crucial impact on patients' possibilities to make their voices heard and participate in care and treatment (Sandman and Munthe 2009; Engström 2008). We will name these ethical perspectives *paternalism, autonomy* and *social inclusion* (see Table 5.1).

The Hippocratic Oath (Hippocrates, n.d.), *the paternalistic perspective,* of 400 BC is one of the first known ethical guidelines for health care. According to the oath, staff should use their skills and knowledge for the benefit of the patient, never do harm and always act only in the patient's best interest. This gives a great responsibility to the professional but the patient has few rights, the only important specified right being confidentiality. The professional plans and decides the treatment, and the patients are expected to comply (Charles, Gafni, and Whelan 1999). This power imbalance is problematic and can in the worst cases lead to decisions that may be perceived as abusive by patients.

After the Second World War, the World Medical Association did strengthen the patient's rights in relation to the health care system by adopting the International Code of Medical Ethics (WMA 1949). A key idea, according to the *autonomy perspective,* is that a competent patient has the right to make a decision about their treatment, whether the decision is beneficial for the patient from a professional perspective or not (Charles, Gafni, and Whelan 1999; Sandman et al. 2012). The professionals can only decide about coercive care

TABLE 5.1   An overview of the three ethical perspectives (a modified table, Pelto-Piri, Engström and Engström, 2013; Pelto-Piri and Kjellin, 2021)

Perspective	Core normative document(s)	Core values highlighted	Decision made by (decision-model)
Paternalism	The Hippocratic Oath	Beneficence Non-maleficent	Professionals (Paternalistic model)
Autonomy	The International Code of Medical Ethics	Autonomy Participation	The informed patient (Informed model)
Social inclusion	The Hawaii, Madrid and Kobe declaration	Reciprocity Social justice	The patient and staff, in association with other stakeholders (Shared model)
	Convention on the Rights of Persons with Disabilities	Freedom from coercive practices	

if the patient lacks decision-competence, has a 'serious mental illness' and if not receiving care would have serious consequences for the patient or others. Autonomy is a core value of medicine and often overrides other values in health care (Beauchamp and Childress 2003; Gaylin and Jennings 2003). This can cause problems for the possibilities to communicate and provide good care in psychiatry. One problem is that the autonomy perspective has a negative view of the possibility for communication between humans. Another problem is that the person is often seen as a single individual and the perspective can ignore the patient's context, like cultural background, family and other important social contacts. A third problem with a strong focus on autonomy is that staff will readily accept a "no" from the patient even though the patient is in great need of care and treatment (Radden 2002; Gaylin, and Jennings 2003).

The third perspective, a *social inclusion perspective*, arises from the declarations of Hawaii (WPA 1983), Madrid (WPA 1996) and Kobe (WASP 2004), as well as the Convention on the Rights of Persons with Disabilities (United Nations 2006). Mutual respect and cooperation are core values in these declarations, staff should work in partnership with patients, their families and other important stakeholders. Patients should have the opportunity to participate in their own care and treatment, working in partnership with the staff to find strategies for handling symptoms and other problems in life. The Declaration of Kobe on the Human Rights of People with Mental Illness (signed by The World Association of Social Psychiatry, World Psychiatric Association and others) concludes that services should "support people with mental illnesses and their families and promote equity, non-discrimination in health policy, and special provisions in health care, education, employment, and housing." (WASP 2004). This demand can be seen as a great focus on social justice (Thornton 2007) and gives staff responsibility to respect the values of the patients (Fulford 2007). Treatment and care should be decided on together with the patient and other stakeholders (Sandman and Munthe 2009). An important aspect of the Kobe Declaration is access to user-friendly services which could minimise detainment and coercion (United Nations 2006; Langley, Wolstenholme and Cooke 2018). This perspective places high demands on staff members, who have to deal with the power imbalance that exists in the relationship with the service users and be responsive to the narratives of users.

These perspectives differ in that the first two are based on ethics that apply to the entire healthcare system, while the social inclusion perspective is developed by psychiatrists' own organisations. These three perspectives are often seen as complementary to each other, but some authors claim that "the biomedical model of mental illness is incompatible with a human right-based approach" (Russo 2020, 152), which indicates that there can be a built-in conflict within the practice and ethics in psychiatry.

2 The User Organisations' Narratives

The Swedish user organisations started as a radical left-wing activist movement in the 1960s, supported by anti-psychiatry intellectuals. The following period was more characterised by user organisations acting like trade unions, moving towards a more democratic work in dialogue with the psychiatric and social services. Today user organisations are more integrated in the mental health system and have become active partners in the co-creation and in co-production of psychiatric services as volunteers or employees. A good example of this is peer-supporters, working with patients as an expert by experience with the support of the user organisation (Table 5.2).

2.1 Institutionalization and Paternalism

Dorothea Dix and many other reformers in the nineteenth century advocated the idea of mental hospitals instead of asylums, prisons or almshouses (Muckenhoupt 2003; Norvoll 2007). The hospital was intended to provide a sheltered place where patients could live and heal rather than being placed in

TABLE 5.2   The Swedish history of psychiatry and the user organisations narratives

Period	Organisational narratives	A typical organisation	A typical slogan
Institutionalization and paternalism	A radical left-wing activism movement	National Association for Social and Mental Health (RSMH)	Away with coercion and oppression in mental health care
Deinstitutionalization and autonomy	Trade union Democratic work	Schizophrenia Association	Nothing about us without us
Transinstitutionalization and social inclusion	Entrepreneurial Co-creation and Co-production	The Swedish Partnership for Mental Health (NSPH)	This is how we want it.

institutions not designed for this group of citizens; instead, their needs should be met in a humane and organised way. Society was going to be a better place to live with institutions like mental hospitals and institutions for persons with intellectual disabilities, drug users and persons with disturbing behaviour. During this time, the focus was on creating a good society for the citizens, but the service users were not asked what support or treatment they preferred, it was a pronounced paternalistic perspective on care and society's obligations.

The Western world saw a large expansion in the number of mental hospitals. In contrast to previous solutions, these institutions were designed to be comfortable places for patients. The mental hospitals fulfilled many needs for people with severe mental distress, which included therapy, medical treatment, work, vocational training, and a sense of community. At the same time, the institutional system contributed to continuous differentiation. People with mental distress, or other behavioural problems, were separated from the 'normal' citizens. In spite of all positive ideals, institutions were often places with poor living conditions, over-crowded, and patients were maltreated and abused. The staff had a dual role: the treatment of patients and the social control of people with abnormal behaviour (Norvoll 2007). The first community-based alternatives were implemented in the 1920s, although the number of institutions continued to increase. In the late 1960s, approximately 35,000 persons with mental distress lived their lives in these institutions in Sweden (Forsberg 1994). At this time, new psychiatric drugs made a major difference for psychiatric care. Patients who had previously been seen as 'wild' with externalised behaviours were now strongly sedated, which made them easier to manage by ward staff, and which reduced the need for coercion.

In the 1960s, citizens who had been detained in institutions such as mental hospitals, residential homes and prisons organised themselves. These user organisations were called R-organisations – the R standing for "justice for the voiceless" (in Swedish the word for 'Justice' is 'Rättvisa'). They reported on abuse and coercion in mental hospitals and other institutions and in the 60s and 70s held an influential voice in the political debates. The R-organisations did a reportage inspired by the German reporter Günter Wallraff, who in 1969 had himself admitted to a mental hospital where he pretended to be an alcoholic. Five Swedish journalists produced an issue of the magazine called *Cared to Insanity: Report from a Swedish Mental Hospital* (Pockettidningen 1975). Three reporters pretended to be 'mentally ill' and were admitted as patients, two reporters got jobs as nurse assistants and a doctor joined them at the same hospital and they reported to the magazine. For a week, they worked undercover before they were revealed as investigators. They got enough inside information about the psychiatric practices, and their article about coercion and the staff behaviour had a great impact on the Swedish discussion about mental hospitals. In the R-organisations' organisational narrative, such words as abuse, oppression and coercion were commonly used, and one slogan was: "Away with coercion and oppression in mental health care." (RSMH, n.d.). New ideas, such as strengthening users' self-determination, was the underlying principle of R-organisations. The mentally distressed should have the same rights, opportunities and obligations as other groups in society. These included the right to service, support, care, and the demand that users' own choices and priorities should be respected. The R-organisations' work can be characterised as left-wing activism. It was conflict-orientated and supported by an intellectual anti-psychiatric trend, as was the case in many other Western countries (Crossley 1999). They had a great impact on the media, and it succeeded in influencing the public narrative of psychiatry, thereby forcing the issue of deinstitutionalization into the political agenda.

2.2 Deinstitutionalization and Autonomy

During the twentieth century there was a trend towards increased democratization. The main motive behind deinstitutionalization was to strengthen the individual's rights and self-determination to live in society, regardless of any obstacles caused by mental distress. In Sweden, the system of institutional psychiatry dominated until the 1980s, when a series of government investigations began to formulate a new policy (SOU 1984; SOU 2006). This new discourse had an emphasis on outpatient care characterised by a holistic approach, easy access and prevention. Service, support and care were going to be provided mainly as outpatient services, in as open forms as possible and in the user's local community. The services' aim was to support the autonomy and integrity of the individual.

Underlying factors for deinstitutionalization have been the development of outpatient-based methodology, new drugs for psychosis, criticism of the conditions at mental hospitals and the considerable costs associated with institutional care. In the late 1980s, the first mental hospitals were closed in Sweden, and the ambition to develop outpatient-based psychiatric services began to result in concrete initiatives. Deinstitutionalization, however, has encountered many difficulties. An early problem was that Sweden had a history of extensive public-driven social and health services built around a strong belief in 'the good state'. It took longer than in most European countries before the ideas of deinstitutionalization and user influence in psychiatry became mainstream in Swedish policy. Another problem was the gap between reduced inpatient care and an underfunded system of community-based care and support. This gap made it difficult to achieve the goals of the reform policy.

At this time, in the late 1980s, many new user organisations with different agendas were formed, and the user movement became more dialogical with politicians and the psychiatric services, they negotiated rather than acted as an activist movement. User organisations started to work more like trade unions seeking influence, and a process of incorporation into the psychiatric health care system started (Eriksson 2015 and 2018). Many of these new organisations, like The Schizophrenia Association, focused on one specific group of diagnoses. They demanded that users be able to participate in their own care. The rhetoric of user involvement at the time was optimistic, promising improved services, conditions and positions for service users, a slogan was "Nothing about us without us" (Brukarföreningarna n.d.). The Schizophrenia Association, but also RSMH and others, were prominent organisations in the work for deinstitutionalization and a more modern psychiatry based on outpatient psychiatric care and support from social services. In this period, user influence increasingly took the form of a central organisational concept at all levels of social and psychiatric services in Sweden (SKL 2010).

2.3   Transinstitutionalisation and Social Inclusion

Since the 90s, the Swedish welfare state, as the rest of Western societies, has undergone an extensive neoliberal transformation. The citizen is now seen as a consumer who has the right to demand services from the system (Esposito 2014). In this neoliberal welfare system, social problems are understood with the help of individualistic explanatory models rather than structural ones. High demands are placed on individuals; they have to be strong consumers who request services and sometimes priority is given to those who are most insistent towards services. A result of this neoliberal turn is that everyone was given a care guarantee; to get a first meeting with the health services within a certain timeframe, regardless of the severity of their needs (SOU 2013). This approach moves resources from seriously distressed users to citizens with less serious distress. Another result of this new discourse was that the public sector no longer had the exclusive right to create, plan and deliver psychiatric services, except for coercive care. This development opened up the possibility for the users' movement to be a partner in co-creation and co-production of psychiatric services (SKR 2015). Sweden's participation in United Nations Agenda 2030 and the 17 sustainable development goals means, among other things, that social innovations should be encouraged and that all groups in society should be able to participate in social life. This is a social inclusion perspective were a human rights-based psychiatry is seen as a tool for developing good psychiatric practice (Broberg et al. 2020).

Deinstitutionalisation has been positive for the majority of patients, with new forms of treatment and care. The lives of chronically and severely mentally distressed persons have sometimes changed from institutionalised living to community living with adequate treatment and support. There are also service users who have experienced a transinstitutionalisation, where large institutions have been replaced with smaller and somewhat more home-like community-based institutions (Topor 1993; Grönberg-Eskel 2012). At the same time a re-institutionalization process has started where former patients from mental hospital have been transferred to other institutions like forensic psychiatry, residential homes or prisons (Priebe et al. 2005).

In order to give the user organisations in Sweden a strong and joint voice in society, The Swedish Partnership for Mental Health (NSPH) was founded in 2007. NSPH is made up of thirteen organisations within the mental health area. All these organisations work with their special focus in the mental health area. NSPH advocates that the voices of people with personal experience of mental distress must be heard, and taken into account, when forming policies and services. The user organisations of today are less conflict-oriented; they seek more consensus with the psychiatric services. NSPH's (2018) desire is a recovery-oriented psychiatry characterised by

- Dignity and empowerment,
- Equality and non-discrimination,
- Participation and transparency.

Earlier, user organisations in the earlier stage sought to influence decisions and radically transform the psychiatric services, now they aim to actively use their competence about recovery. They demand to be a partner and be involved in co-creation and co-production of psychiatric services. A slogan has been "This is how we want it to be." (NSPH 2018). The user organisations have become an integral part in the creation and production of psychiatric care (SKL 2011; SKL 2015) and many former service users have an income from the psychiatric services or projects funded by government agencies. They might work with peer support or have other functions in these psychiatric services. Some are more 'entrepreneurial', selling their services as lecturers, by talking about their own and others' experiences of mental health issues. NSPH receives grants for projects to develop new methods and innovations for the psychiatric services. This cooperation has produced tendencies towards co-option of user organisations (Eriksson 2018). Co-option occurs since there is an imbalance of power between psychiatric services and the user's organisations. A co-opting process gives user organisations an opportunity to influence the decision-making, but at the same time, it can neutralise oppositional user representatives and adapt them into the psychiatric organisation. There is a risk of psychiatrization which means that the user representatives start to internalise the psychiatric organisations interests, understanding and goals; starting to tell the "right narrative" in order to be accepted by professionals and policymakers (Eriksson 2018; Logan and Karter 2022).

Some of the projects driven by user organisations are successful examples of co-creation and co-production, like "The national suicide helpline". The origin for the project was that Mind, a user organisation, saw a lack in the psychiatric services' work with suicide prevention around 2010. The suicide prevention was not successful, and the suicide rate in Sweden was increasing in some age groups. Something was missing, and discussions in Mind led to the desire to create a new service to make a difference. There was a need for a dialogue that was not a professional meeting but rather a meeting without the inevitable power imbalances contained in this type of conversation. The kind of dialogue they saw a need for was more characterised by fellow human compassion, empathy, and charity. They agreed that there was a need for a 24-hour telephone helpline open for people in need where volunteering fellow users and others were going to answer the calls. The telephone helpline was implemented in 2015.

3 Is Psychiatry Moving from Paternalism to Social Inclusion?

The user organisations' work to transform psychiatry has been successful in many ways. The most obvious change is that the large mental hospitals characterised by hard paternalism are closed and most patients are more integrated in society. Deinstitutionalization and increased access to health care have improved the quality of life for many persons suffering from serious mental distress. We can also see a greater transparency in psychiatric services today, compared to earlier, which enables new forms of cooperation. It is more common today to really listen to the patient's own voice, which allows for a more person-centred care. Despite these successes, some problems still need to be addressed in order for service users to be socially included. Major difficulties are: 1) the lack of support to the most severely mentally distressed users, 2) old and new forms of coercion and 3) co-option of the user organisations.

The lack of support for the most severe mentally distressed users is a major concern. As argued, the deinstitutionalization of psychiatry became a transinstitutionalisation for many users with serious mental distress, who just moved from large institutions to smaller ones. Others, who were not assessed to have as great a need for support, did not receive community-based housing. In these cases, the right to autonomy often overruled the safety and well-being of the user and allowed them to be "dying with one's rights on her lips" (Treffert 2006). It is easy to be critical of transinstitutionalisation, still, we cannot fully depend on outpatient psychiatric care. More housing with various degrees of supervision and facilities with a full range of services needs to be a part of the mental health services. The mental health services of communities have not been able to start enough specialised teams, such as assertive outreach and early intervention teams, to meet the needs of service users. Another problem is that evidence-based methods are seldom used by the practitioners in community settings, which might have contributed to the failure to address the needs of users. A new generation of users with severe mental distress can end up in poverty; as homeless, substance users or criminals and present a major challenge to social and psychiatric services (Turnpenny et al. 2018). The failure to address the needs of users has led to excess mortality; mentally distressed persons are at risk of dying 15–20 years earlier than the general population in Sweden (Wahlbeck et al. 2011). As a reaction to these problems, a re-institutionalization of users has taken place. Many users with severe psychiatric distress are faced with being institutionalised in forensic psychiatry, residential homes or prisons. This process has occurred largely unnoticed by the public and with little professional or public debate.

Old and new forms of coercion are exercised side by side by the psychiatric services today. The old form of coercion still exists, psychiatric patients or survivors of psychiatry, continue to testify about coercive measure, detainment, abusive treatment, maladministration and lack of support, and some employees report poor working conditions and insufficient patient safety (Turnpenny et al. 2018). Apart from legally decided coercive care and measures, patients and staff are reporting on coercion that does not have legal support, so-called perceived or informal coercion (O'Donoghue et al. 2014; Valenti et al. 2015). Users have difficulties to resist this kind of coercion since they are aware of the legal right of psychiatric system to use coercion if they consider it necessary. Despite a contemporary trend towards outpatient care and social inclusion there is simultaneously a trend towards more coercion. A new form of coercion, namely community treatment orders, are being used internationally in psychiatry despite the fact that the intervention seems to be ineffective (Rugkåsa 2016). Community treatment orders have also been implemented in Sweden in 2008. The new law resulted in shorter care episodes in coercive care in inpatient care, but the total number of days with coercion, in inpatient and outpatient care, was increased (Kjellin and Pelto-Piri 2014). In the past, the user organisations were fighting against hard paternalism. Now there is a need to be vigilant that coercion should not be overused in psychiatric services. At the same time, there is still a need and justification for soft paternalism. Coercive care and measures challenge human rights but they are sometimes needed to protect a person's life and dignity. It is far more controversial to defend the view that it is never appropriate to practise soft paternalism or coercion in psychiatry, on the contrary, it is a neglect to leave a psychotic patient alone if the patient can be helped by treatment and/or support. To reduce coercive measures several interventions can be used. A literature review indicates that awareness among staff that coercive measures can be traumatic, and that care should not cause harm, decreases the use of coercive measures (Gooding 2018). Another intervention is care based on respect for human rights; it supports personal recovery and reduces coercive measures. There are also evidence-based interventions such as Safewards and Six Core Strategies that have proven effective in reducing coercive measures (Gooding 2018; Fernández-Costa 2020). These interventions are rarely used in Sweden.

Co-option of user organisations is a great risk since user influence is about making a difference. It is relevant to acknowledge that user organisations have a narrative to tell which represents an alternative to the psychiatric discourse; a right-based perspective rather than the biomedical model. An overarching question about user influence is whether it is a matter of fundamentally changing the services, or if it is to adjust them to work more optimally and not addressing for example, power structures, attitudes or treatment. A user influence that leads to a radical change of psychiatric services requires that users, possibly in cooperation with internal change agents and other citizens, can mobilise a sufficiently powerful position. User organisations have seldom enforced major changes in the psychiatric services by themselves. Most often, they have had modest influence in the final decision-making (Eriksson 2018), but co-option of a user organisation is not necessarily a sign of failure (Eriksson 2015). The important aspect is to what extent the user organisation is able to maintain self-determination and act independently despite co-option.

Finally, we want to ask whether psychiatry is moving from paternalism to social inclusion? As we have shown above numerous examples which suggest that psychiatry is on the road to social inclusion. The users and their organisations have gone from being oppositional in society to being an integral part of the psychiatric health care system. Still there are problems, like the ones presented above: most importantly, the lack of support for the most severely mentally distressed users and the use of coercion in the psychiatric services. These problems need to be addressed at the policy level rather than within the psychiatric health care system (Forbes and Sashidharan 1997). Who, if not the user organisations, have the best conditions for representing the most vulnerable users and drawing the public's attention to coercive practices? To do so, there is a lot to learn from history, where user organisations have approached their aims like activists and resembled tough trade-union representatives. To be able to address these problems, it is important not to be fully co-opted into the psychiatric services and into projects funded by government agencies. More than ever, free user organisations are needed that can give a voice to those who are unable to argue for their rights themselves. Then, maybe, we can move towards social inclusion – a society where we are "Leaving No One Behind" (United Nations 2016).

References

Beauchamp, Tom L., and James F. Childress. 2003. *Principles of Biomedical Ethics*. 6th ed. New York: Oxford University Press.

Broberg, Emma, Agneta Persson, Anna Jacobson, and Anna-Karin Engqvist. 2020. "A Human Rights-Based Approach to Psychiatry: Is It Possible?" *Health Hum Rights* 22: 121–131. https://www.ncbi.nlm.nih.gov/pmc/articles/PMC7348414/pdf/hhr-22-01 -121.pdf.

Brukarföreningarna. n.d. https://www.brukarforeningarna.se/.

Charles, Cathy, Amiram Gafni, and Tim Whelan. 1999. "Decision-Making in the Physician-Patient Encounter: Revisiting the Shared Treatment Decision-Making Model." *Social Science and Medicine* 49, no. 5: 651–61. http://ac.els-cdn.com/S027795 3699001458/1-s2.0-S0277953699001458-main.pdf?_tid=7d00fc9c-ab5d-11e3 -8f50-00000aacb362&acdnat=1394790557_79223ced0787c49798be45e7b2ec7f88.

Crossley, Nick. 1999. "Fish, Field, Habitus and Madness: the First Wave Mental Health Users Movement in Great Britain." *British Journal of Sociology 50*, no. 4: 647–670.

Engström, Karin. 2008. *Delaktighet under tvång* [In Swedish]. PhD diss., Örebro: Örebro University.

Eriksson, Erik. 2015. *Sanktionerat motstånd: Brukarinflytande som fenomen och praktik.* [In Swedish]. Lunds Universitet, Socialhögskolan.

Eriksson, Erik. 2018. "Four features of Cooptation – User Involvement as Sanctioned Resistance." *Nordic Welfare Research* 3, no. 1: 7–17. DOI:10.18261/issn.2464-4161-2018 -01-02.

Esposito, Luigi, and Fernando M. Perez. 2014. "Neoliberalism and the Commodification of Mental Health." *Humanity & Society* 38, no. 4: 414–42. https://doi.org /10.1177/0160597614544958.

Fernández-Costa, Damián, Juan Gómez-Salgado, Javier Fagundo-Rivera, Jorge Martín-Pereira, Blanca Prieto-Callejero and Juan Jesús García-Iglesias. 2020. "Alternatives to the Use of Mechanical Restraints in the Management of Agitation or Aggressions of Psychiatric Patients: A Scoping Review." *Journal of Clinical Medicine,* 9 (9): 2791. DOI: https://doi.org/10.3390/jcm9092791.

Forbes, Joan, and Sashi P. Sashidharan. 1997. "User Involvement in Services – Incorporation or Challenge?" *British Journal of Social Work* 27, no 4. https://doi.org/10.1093/oxfordjournals.bjsw.a011237.

Fredriksson, Anna, and Åsa Moberg. 2020. *De omöjliga – Från psykiatrireform till dyr och dålig vård.* [In Swedish] Stockholm: Natur och Kultur.

Forsberg, Erik. 1994. *Den stora utflyttningen – studier av psykiatrins omvandling.* Skriftserie, Socialt arbete. Göteborg: Göteborgs Universitet.

Fulford, Bill. 2004. "Ten Principles of Values-Based Medicine." In *The Philosophy of Psychiatry: A Companion,* edited by Jenifer Radden, 205–234. New York: Oxford University Press.

Fulford, Bill, Tim Thornton, and Gregory Graham. 2007. *Oxford Textbook of Philosophy and Psychiatry.* Oxford: Oxford University Press.

Gaylin, Willard, and Bruce Jennings. 2003. *The Perversion of Autonomy. Coercion and Constraints in a Liberal Society.* Washington DC: Georgetown University Press.

Gooding, Piers, Bernadette McSherry, Cath Roper, and Flick Grey. 2018. *Alternatives to Coercion in Mental Health Settings: A Literature Review.* Commissioned by the United Nations Office at Geneva to inform the report of the United Nations Special Rapporteur on the Rights of Persons with Disabilities. Melbourne Social Equity Institute. https://socialequity.unimelb.edu.au/__data/assets/pdf_file/0012/2898525/Alternatives-to-Coercion-Literature-Review-Melbourne-Social-Equity-Institute.pdf.

Grönberg, Eskel M. 2012. *Från slutna institutioner till institutionaliserat omhändertagande.* Karlstad: Karlstad University Studies.

Hippocrates, n.d. *The Hippocratic Oath.* https://en.wikipedia.org/wiki/Hippocratic_Oath.

Kemp, Wolfgang. 1996. "Narrative." In *Critical Terms for Art History,* edited by Robert S. Nelson and Richard Schiff, 2nd ed., 62–75. Chicago and London: The University of Chicago Press.

Kjellin, Lars, and Veikko Pelto-Piri. 2014. "Community Treatment Orders in a Swedish County – Applied as Intended? *BMC Research Notes,* 7: 879. https://doi.org/10.1186/1756-0500-7-879.

Langley, Joe, Daniel Wolstenholme, and Jo Cooke. 2018. "Collective Making as Knowledge Mobilisation: the Contribution of Participatory Design in the Co-Creation of Knowledge in Healthcare." *BMC Health Services Research 18,* no. 1: 585. https://doi.org/10.1186/s12913-018-3397-y.

Logan, Jenny, and Justin M. Karter. 2022. "Psychiatrization of Resistance: The Co-option of Consumer, Survivor, and Ex-patient Movements in the Global South." *Frontiers in Sociology 7,* Article 784390. https://doi:10.3389/fsoc.2022.784390.

Muckenhoupt, Margaret. 2003. *Dorothea Dix: Advocate for Mental Health Care.* New York: Oxford University Press.

Norvoll, Reidun. 2007. *Det lukkede rum. Bruk av skjerming som behandling og kontroll i psykiatriske akuttposter.* Thesis. Oslo: Universitetet Oslo.

NSPH. 2018. *Så vill vi ha det - inget om oss utan oss.* http://nsph.se/wp-content/uploads/2018/06/NSPH-Sa-vill-vi-ha-det.pdf.

O'Donoghue, Brian, Eric Roche, Stephan Shannon, John Lyne, Kevin Madigan, and Larkin Feeney. 2014. "Perceived Coercion in Voluntary Hospital Admission." *Psychiatry Res* 215, no. 1: 120–126. https://doi.org/10.1016/j.psychres.2013.10.016.

Pelto-Piri, Veikko. 2015. *Ethical Considerations in Psychiatric Inpatient Care: The Ethical Landscape in Everyday Practice as Described by Staff* [Dissertation]. Örebro *Studies in Medicine 120.* Örebro University.

Pelto-Piri, Veikko, Karin Engström, and Ingemar Engström. 2013. "Paternalism, Autonomy and Reciprocity: Ethical Perspectives in Encounters with Patients in Psychiatric In-Patient care." *BMC Medical Ethics*, 14: 49. DOI: 10.1186/1472-6939-14-49.

Pelto-Piri, Veikko, and Lars Kjellin. 2021. "Social Inclusion and the Prevention of Violence. A Qualitative Interview Study with Service Users, Staff Members and Ward Managers." *BMC Health Services Research*, 21: 1255. https://doi.org/10.1186/s12913-021-07178-6

Pockettidningen R. 1975. *Vårdad till vanvett: rapport från ett svenskt mentalsjukhus.* Stockholm: Prisma.

Priebe, Stefan, Alli Badesconyi, Angelo Fioritti, Lars Hansson, Reinhold Kilian, Francisco Torres-Gonzales, Trevor Turner, and Durk Wiersma. 2005. "Reinstitutionalisation in Mental Health Care: Comparison of Data on Service Provision from Six European Countries." *BMJ* 330 no. 7483: 123–126. DOI: https://doi.org/10.1136/bmj.38296.611215.AE.

Radden, Jennifer. 2002. "Psychiatric Ethics." *Bioethics* 16, no. 5: 397–411.

Rugkåsa, Jorun. 2016. "Effectiveness of Community Treatment Orders: The International Evidence". *Canadian Journal of Psychiatry. Revue canadienne de psychiatrie* 61, no. 1:15–24. https://journals.sagepub.com/doi/10.1177/0706743715620415.

Russo, Jasna, and Stephanie Wooley. 2020. "The Implementation of the Convention on the Rights of Persons with Disabilities: More Than Just Another Reform of Psychiatry." *Health Hum Rights* 22, no. 1:151–161. https://www.ncbi.nlm.nih.gov/pmc/articles/PMC7348441/pdf/hhr-22-01-151.pdf.

RSMH. n.d. http://rsmh.se/wp-content/uploads/2018/10/REV_1605_TIDSLINJE.pdf.

Sadler, John Z. 2004. *Values and Psychiatric Diagnosis.* Oxford: Oxford University Press.

Sandman, Lars, Bradi B. Granger, Inger Ekman, and Christian Munthe. 2021. "Adherence, Shared Decision-Making and Patient Autonomy." *Med Health Care Philos* 15, no. 2: 115–127. https://doi.org/10.1007/s11019-011-9336-x.

Sandman, Lars, and Chistian Munthe. 2009. "Shared Decision-Making and Patient Autonomy." *Theor Med Bioeth* 30, no. 4: 289–310. https://doi.org/10.1007/s11017-009-9114-4.

SKL. 2010. *Patient – och brukarmedverkan. Positioneringspapper – För ökad kvalitet och effektivitet i hälso- och sjukvård och socialtjänst.* Stockholm: Sveriges kommuner och landsting.

SKL. 2011. *Brukarmedverkan. Ett nytt sätt att arbete.* Stockholm: Sveriges kommuner och landsting.

SKL. 2015. *När brukare och patienter blir medskapare.* Stockholm: Sveriges kommuner och landsting.

Socialstyrelsen. 2018. *Nationella riktlinjer för vård och stöd vid schizofreni och schizofreniliknande tillstånd. 2018–9–6.* Socialstyrelsen.

Thornton, Tim. 2007. *Essential Philosophy of psychiatry.* Oxford: Oxford University Press.

SOU 1984:64. Psykiatrin, tvånget och rättssäkerheten: betänkande av Socialberedningen. Stockholm: LiberTryck.

SOU 2006:100. Ambition och ansvar. Nationell strategi för utveckling av samhällets insatser till personer med psykiska sjukdomar och funktionshinder. Socialdepartementet. https://www.regeringen.se/49b6aa/contentassets/c128c16b19a94dc6ab997 68cbb8176dd/ambition-och-ansvar.-nationell-strategi-for-utveckling-av -samhallets-insatser-till-personer-med-psykiska-sjukdomar-och-funktionshinder -sou-2006100.

SOU 2013:2. Patientlag. Stockholm: Socialdepartementet https://www.regeringskansliet .se/contentassets/93a9c6ee50fe49a183aab8389997b7f7/patientlag---delbetan kande-av-patientmaktsutredningen-sou-20132.

Stacey, Gemma, Anne Felton, Alastair Morgan, Theo Stickley, Martin Willis, Bob Diamond, Philip Houghton, Beverley Johnson, and John Dumenya. 2016. "A Critical Narrative Analysis of Shared Decision-Making in Acute Inpatient Mental Health Care." *J Interprof Care* 30, no. 1: 35–41. https://doi.org/10.3109/13561820.2015.1064878.

Topor, Alain. 1993. *Vad hjälper? Vägar till återhämtning från svåra psykiska problem.* Natur & Kultur. Stockholm.

Treffert, Donald A. 2006. "Dying with Their Rights On." *American Journal of Psychiatry* 130 (9): 1041. DOI: 10.1176/ajp.130.9.1041.

Turnpenny, Agnes, Gabor Petri, Ailbhe Finn, Julie Beadle-Brown, and Maria Nyman. 2018. *Mapping and Understanding Exclusion: Institutional, Coercive and Community-Based Services and Practices across Europe.* Brussels, Belgium: Mental Health Europe. https://doi.org/10.22024/UniKent/01.02/64970.

United Nations. 2006. *Convention on the Rights of Persons with Disabilities.* New York: UN, Department of Economic & Social Affairs. https://www.un.org/development /desa/disabilities/convention-on-the-rights-of-persons-with-disabilities.html.

United Nations. 2016. Leaving No One Behind: The Imperative of Inclusive Development. In *Report on the World Social Situation 2016, ST/ESA/362.* New York: UN, Department of Economic & Social Affairs. https://www.un.org/esa/socdev/rwss /2016/full-report.pdf

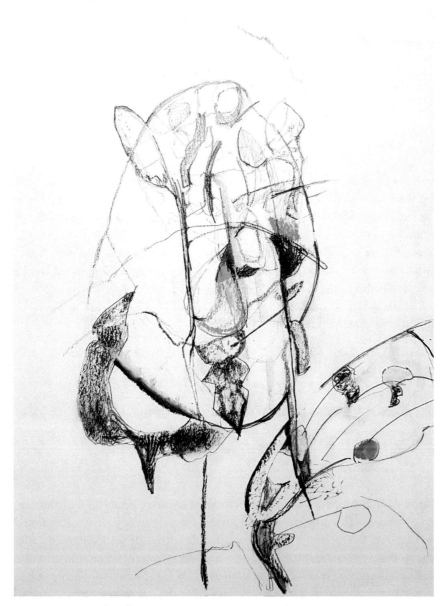

FIGURE 5.1   Marta Wandt

CHAPTER 6

Plaques, Politics and Preservation: Publicly Memorialising Mad People's Labour History

Geoffrey Reaume

Abstract

Activist efforts to preserve and publicly memorialise nineteenth century patient built boundary walls at the former Toronto Asylum for the Insane will be analysed in the context of critically re-interpreting an asylum's past while working with psychiatric facility administrators to ensure this material history is not destroyed and patients' labour history is properly acknowledged. Issues around co-option of this history by psychiatrists as well as some historians' reaction against activist efforts will be critiqued by discussing the politics of memorialising marginalized groups in history and how these efforts challenge traditional interpretations, in this case, mad peoples' unpaid work as exploitation rather than therapy.

Keywords

Mad Peoples' labour history – public history – psychiatric survivor archives – Toronto

1 Introduction

Throughout the nineteenth to mid-twentieth centuries, insane asylum inmates in Canada toiled for no pay under the guise of "moral therapy". Ostensibly aimed to "improve" the mental health of mad people with light work and recreation, "moral therapy" ended up becoming a massive system of economic exploitation of inmates in asylums whereby "therapy" became a cover for using public inmates primarily to build, clean and maintain the day to day physical operation of mental institutions. Asylum operators in nineteenth-century Ontario made no secret of how much money they saved public works by having insane asylum inmates do work for no cost. Indeed, when eastern and western portions of the boundary walls, which are the focus of this article, were reconstructed in 1888–89, Toronto Asylum superintendent, Daniel Clark wrote that the use of inmates in building these walls caused "tens of thousands of dollars saved" to the provincial government (Annual Report 1890, 42–43). The Toronto Asylum at 999 Queen St. West was originally opened in 1850 (a temporary asylum had operated three miles east of this site from 1841–1850) where to this day a mental health facility continues to operate in what is now a very heavily populated area of the city just west of the downtown core. Asylum inmates built the first stone wall surrounding 50 acres of the asylum property in 1860. However, the east and west walls had to be torn down and re-built in 1889 as urbanisation encroached on the once pastoral setting so that the property was reduced to 26 acres by this time, dimensions which still exist today, over 130 years later (Reaume 2006, 74, 85).

Between 1970 and 1975, the old asylum buildings and all of the north boundary wall were demolished to make way for new buildings which eventually officially opened in 1979 (Court 2000, 194–196). All that exists today of the old nineteenth-century Toronto Asylum are the east, west and south boundary walls, along with two brick workshop/storage buildings in the back (south side) of the property. The front of the property is on Queen Street, one of Toronto's main streets, which faces north; the east wall runs along Shaw Street, a busy thoroughfare. By the early 2000s, there were plans to re-make the entire site again during which there was talk of tearing down the boundary walls, particularly the most visible and well-preserved wall along the east side of this property – the Shaw Street Wall. By this time, I had discovered in my research for my 1997 doctoral dissertation in History at the University of Toronto, published as a book in 2000, that the boundary walls had been built by asylum inmates (Reaume 2000a, 147). Previous to this, the emphasis on preserving the walls, as in the 1970s, had been because they represented the work of a well-known Toronto architect, Kivas Tully. Indeed, as late as 1996, the same year in which I found the information that patients built the wall in publicly accessible annual reports in the Archives of Ontario, a City of Toronto Heritage Report, extolled the importance of the wall's architect to the city's past. This same report claimed that the actual builders of the walls were "none found" (City of Toronto Bylaw No. 1997–0085, Schedule "B" 1996: 3). This was stated, even though the public documents which clearly indicated who toiled on the walls were available only a few blocks away from where this report was produced.

Thus, while local historical preservationists had advocated saving the wall since the 1970s – and were successful in doing so during the reconstruction done on this site during that decade – this was done by their emphasis on the architectural history of this structure designed by a well-known local architect rather than its worth as evidence of the social history of patients who built it and who lived and died behind it. By the time the next major reconstruction started being discussed three decades later and the existence of the boundary walls was threatened yet again, the emphasis shifted significantly due to the active involvement of psychiatric survivors in the preservation and interpretation efforts. This change in emphasis was brought about by a group of people involved in efforts to promote our own history as psychiatric survivors, mad activists or whichever term individuals chose. As a an ex-psychiatric patient who was involved both as an academic historian and activist in researching our past, and wanting to get it out in the wider community to whom it belonged beyond the ivory tower, much of what follows in this article is based on my research.[1] Due to being directly involved in both locating and writing about the original archival sources which documented asylum inmates' labour history, as well as in publicizing this information in a variety of ways with a group of fellow activists over more than a decade covered by this article, much of what follows is an activist account, as much as it is scholarly. As a result, a good deal of this chapter is self-referential since it is intended to explain how one academically trained historian, working with members of the psychiatric survivor/mad community and allies, sought to memorialise exploited insane asylum inmate labourers whose history had not previously been publicly acknowledged since the late 1800s. This chapter is therefore, one example of how public history was undertaken involving multiple participants, the challenges experienced along the way, and the manner in which these efforts have also seen a backlash by some who prefer a more conservative interpretation of this past which, rather than critiquing dominant economic and social relations in asylums, seeks to undermine and distort such interpretations.

When reflecting upon this history it is important to consider how this topic fits into the overall theme of narrating the heritage of psychiatry. Narratives in psychiatric history have only recently begun to include the views of mad people themselves (Reaume 2017). It is therefore not surprising that such views are not reflected in public historical markers which this author has observed with public plaques located at former asylums in Canada, the United States and England. Only with recent activist histories have such efforts changed this narrative approach where public history plaques acknowledge the lives of deceased asylum inmates, as Pemina Yellow Bird has shown regarding Indigenous inmates

---

1   In the interests of what academics refer to as "positionality", it is important to note that I was never a psychiatric patient at the Toronto facility which is the focus of this article. I was a psychiatric in-patient in mental health facilities in Windsor, Ontario (1976) and St. Thomas, Ontario (1979) for a total of six months and was an out-patient in Windsor from 1976–83. I began to be involved in Toronto's psychiatric survivor community in 1990 and remained active until 2013.

buried on the grounds of a closed American asylum (Yellow Bird 2004). In so doing, the concept of narrative – of story-telling – is approached as memory retrieving. At some point in this past, a large number of people would have known that asylum inmates built the boundary walls which are the focus of this chapter. Not only asylum staff and fellow asylum inmates who were alive at the time of this construction and reconstruction, but local residents in the area would have seen this work with their own eyes. That this unpaid inmates' labour was recorded in a public document at all, long before it was buried in an archive, indicates the normalization of how such work was viewed and that it was not always hidden but publicly acknowledged and even boasted about by asylum officials. As the decades wore on, this public knowledge died with those who did the work, or who witnessed and wrote about it in annual reports in documents that were packed off to the archives. While this labour history has not always been buried or forgotten, accounts about the asylum in which it happened, as described in this chapter, until the late 1990s, remained silent about what had been known and publicly documented over one hundred years before. Narratives are not static, they change over time, or are forgotten as people die and documents which, if they mention such marginalized peoples' histories at all, are lost, destroyed or are stored where only a historical researcher might come across them long afterwards. In retrieving such memories from historical documents, the purpose is to ensure that narrative restoration contributes to changing wider stories about the people who lived and died behind these walls. It is also intended to advocate for the physical preservation of difficult parts of our past which resonate today with people in various ways. As Elizabeth Punzi has noted "patients' experiences are difficult to acknowledge when traces of history are erased." (Punzi 2019, 243). Preservation leads to tangible historical reminders if such structures are publicly acknowledged. In doing so, efforts to preserve and mark asylum inmate's historical sites fits into a narrative approach which ensures that the perspectives of mad people are at the forefront of such public commemorations.

2   The Commemorative Site: the Campaign to Preserve and
        Memorialise the Patient-Built Wall-Plaques

The historical importance of this site is that it is one of the last remaining physical symbols of unpaid patient labour from the Toronto Asylum, in this case, a particularly evocative symbol in that patients were made to build the very walls behind which they were confined. The 1860 south wall is also notable for

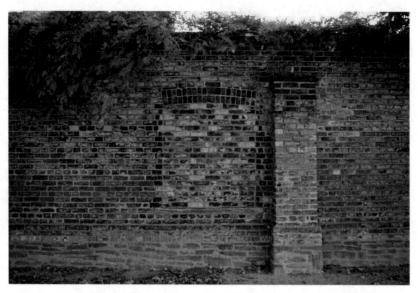

FIGURE 6.1   Geoffrey Reaume, oldest section of the patient built toronto asylum wall
from 1860

not only is it the oldest part of the former provincial asylum still in existence, it
also is the oldest example of patients' labour anywhere in Ontario.[2]

Since 1998, public history events within the psychiatric survivor community in Toronto have focused on using the patient-built wall as a site of both
commemoration and public education. The first efforts to publicize the labour
history of the wall were in the form of a play which was performed at various times between 1998 and 2000, at two venues right next to the property
where the wall is situated, as well as once in the psychiatric facility itself. This
play, *Angels of 999*, was written, produced and acted almost entirely (though
not exclusively) by psychiatric survivors, including people who were public as
current and former patients at this psychiatric facility. It was based on research
from my PhD dissertation and used the words and experiences of historical
patients as was revealed by archival records.[3] The patient-built wall was *the*

---

2   The next oldest surviving example in the province of a building built by insane asylum inmates
is from 1861 in Amherstburg, Ontario at the former Malden Asylum. See: Reaume 2006, 76.

3   The initial drafts of this play were written by myself and were then dramaturged by Ruth
Stackhouse and Ken Innes of Friendly Spike Theatre Band, and additional script contributions were made by members of the theatre troupe. It was workshopped over a weekend
of performances in June 1998, and then performed for 10 days in May 1999 and for two
weeks in April 2000, along with several shows at different venues during this time, the last
performance being in July 2000. The book launch for *Remembrance of Patients Past* in April

central motif in the play around which the actors performed, with unpaid labour being a major theme of the play. For the first time since nineteenth century annual reports mentioned them, the building of the wall with unpaid patients' labour was publicly acknowledged. One psychiatric survivor, who was then a member of the Queen Street Patients Council, told me after seeing the play that she had never thought much about the wall before but now she looks at it quite differently and with some pride knowing that patients were the ones who built it. It was with this sense of pride, and also righteous indignation that this history had been so wilfully ignored for so long, along with the exploitation it represents of unpaid labour and contempt for the contributions of mad people to our past, that this play catapulted the history of the wall into further venues for public history.

Just as the run of the play was ending, another form of getting the word out about this history was beginning – wall tours. During these tours, the lives, deaths and unpaid work of the men and women who were patients at the old asylum are described near the places where they once toiled as represented by the boundary walls they built, lived and worked behind (Reaume 2010–11). By re-casting the stones of oppression and exclusion as stones whose stories can liberate forgotten histories and include people in our collective remembrances who had previously been forgotten, this wall of confinement was used as a tool for mad people's history that would otherwise not be available if it were torn down. Much as I respect the views of psychiatric survivors who argued for the demolition of the wall, I disagreed with their argument that by tearing down the wall stigma will somehow be torn down with it. It is prejudices in people's minds that create discrimination not the bricks from this old wall. If this visible symbol of past exploitation and oppression were to be torn down, we will only succeed in eradicating part of our own past that must be dealt with and which will be all the more difficult to have publicly addressed and acknowledged if it does not exist by being right in front of us where it cannot be avoided. As time went on, the widespread support in the psychiatric survivor and mad communities in Toronto, including from some who previously wanted the boundary walls and all physical reminders of the old asylum demolished, was central to ensuring not only the preservation of the structure but interpreting this site from the perspectives of mad people's history. It would have been impossible to have accomplished this task without wider community involvement and help which was built up over a decade of activist efforts. It was not and could

---

2000 was centred around the play and, before the play, we went out of the theatre to the nearby west wall where we toasted the wall and all the patients who built it and who lived and died behind it.

not have been a solo effort by any one person. Preserving this wall as a heritage site, which is governed by a bylaw between the existing hospital and the City of Toronto, is essential to the practical preservation of mad people's public history and its contemporary relevance well into the future.

3   The Historical Site of Contention: Cracks in the Wall 2000–2007

All of this leads to the debates around how to preserve and interpret the history of this wall since the early 2000s. When plans for the redevelopment of the former Toronto Asylum site, now called the *Centre for Addiction and Mental Health* (CAMH) started to be discussed, the fate of the patient-built wall was also raised. At the launch for my book on patients' history on this site on April 14, 2000, just after we toasted the wall and the patients who built it and who lived and died behind it, a CAMH consultant asked me what I thought was going to happen to that wall (motioning to the west wall where we were standing). I said it should be preserved as a memorial to the patients who built it. The person who asked me this did not say what was going to happen to those old walls that day, but did indicate its future was not clear, especially as some people saw the wall as representing stigma. By 2001, there was more talk making the rounds that the east wall along Shaw Street would be torn down – this is the most visible of all the existing walls to passersby in vehicles or pedestrians. That same year, the Psychiatric Survivor Archives, Toronto (PSAT) was founded and members advocated preserving this structure, beginning in late 2001 with letters and attendance at meetings the following year. By 2003, these efforts led to a public "Open Ideas Competition" sponsored by the Centre for Addiction and Mental Health and the City of Toronto about what to do with the east wall. In the midst of this competition the Psychiatric Survivor Archives initiated and organized a "Town Hall on this Historic Wall" a term thought up by archives' member Graeme Bacque; there were eventually 127 entries and agreement that the east wall would be preserved, along with the rest of the boundary walls.[4] The term "Town Hall" is used in North America to refer to a public gathering held for interested members of a community to discuss a topic of concern – in this case, a meeting about what to do with the nineteenth century Toronto Asylum patient-built walls.

---

4   The headline of an article about the PSAT organized Town Hall gives an idea of the pessimism then surrounding the fate of the east wall: Chris Sorensen, "Future of Shaw Street Wall in Doubt", *Toronto Star*, February 13, 2003. The two designs which won the competition were not implemented. This design competition was separate from PSAT's wall plaques' campaign, though it was part of the new public history awareness surrounding the patient built wall.

Beginning in 2004, meetings began to be held with PSAT representatives, staff from the Empowerment Council at CAMH, archivists and hospital staff, all of whom met along with architects who specialize in preserving historical structures. The architects pin-pointed the areas of the wall, primarily on the west side, that were in need of most immediate conservation. In 2007, two CAMH "clients" were employed on this preservation work in an agreement with the construction company and building trades union. PSAT recommended in

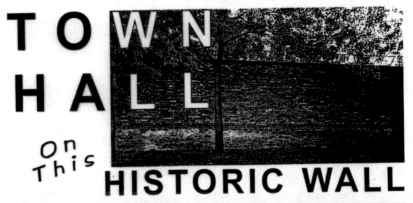

TOWN HALL

on This HISTORIC WALL

Do you have Ideas about what to do with this historic wall that runs along Shaw at Queen?

Built by Toronto Asylum inmate labourers in the late 1800s, there are plans afoot to re-develop this wall along with the rest of the Centre for Addiction and Mental Health site, 1001 Queen Street West. An "Open Ideas Competition" run by CAMH and the City of Toronto Heritage Preservation Services is taking place right now to get input from the public. Time is short as the competition ends March 31 - What do you think should be done with the Shaw Street Wall?

People familiar with urban planning, local history and the "Open Ideas Competition" process will be at this meeting to provide background information and answer questions.

Public Meeting at

PARKDALE LIBRARY
1303 QUEEN ST. W.
WEDNESDAY, FEBRUARY 12
6 PM - 8 PM

Light refreshments will be served

for more information call (416) 324-8808
or e-mail <info@psychiatricsurvivorarchives.com>
**Sponsored by Psychiatric Survivor Archives, Toronto
and Parkdale Community Legal Services**
http://www.psychiatricsurvivorarchives.com

FIGURE 6.2   Graeme Bacque, Town Hall on this Historic Wall, February 12, 2003

June 2004 that, when conservation work commenced, people who are "clients" of the current facility should be employed at good union wages to work on preserving what is, after all, their history, unlike the original workers who were paid nothing. This was agreed to by the various parties by 2006, and the next summer saw this paid work done on preserving the west wall.

A second Town Hall on the Wall was organized by PSAT and the Empowerment Council in March 2005. At this meeting, architects presented ideas about preserving the wall and psychiatric survivors and community members voiced their views. The important point to emphasize is that psychiatric survivors were involved throughout this process in which preserving the wall was secured and implemented. This preservation work did not always turn out the way PSAT had advocated – a small but perfectly preserved portion of the east wall at the south end of the property was dismantled to make way for widening a road in 2007. Nevertheless, these dismantled bricks were re-used on the west wall's preservation work in summer 2007, which was a consolation of sorts; a further small portion of the east wall was removed in 2019 for a road. These efforts to preserve the wall were a collaborative effort involving the Psychiatric Survivor Archives the Empowerment Council, CAMH, the CAMH Archives and administration along with the City of Toronto and architectural firms. This alliance between such diverse groups, while tense at times given the different perspectives on the history of the site and the past and present practices of psychiatry, nevertheless produced an important outcome for respecting mad people's history.

Right from the beginning of advocating for the preservation of the patient built walls in 2001–2002, PSAT promoted the idea of public markers to acknowledge the labour and social history of the asylum inmates which these walls shadowed for so very long. After the preservation of the walls was assured in 2004, work next turned to wording for potential plaques. In the summer of 2005, texts for eight different plaques to go up at different sites around the wall, were written by myself, approved by the PSAT Board and endorsed by the CAMH Archives which also added some minor revisions. The wording for each of these eight plaque texts focused on different aspects of patient labour and social history on the site and follow stops along the wall tour route. It was important to ensure that each plaque should be located near a particular place of historical importance associated with the descriptive text. This text was provided to the CAMH administration at a meeting in February 2006 and was raised at subsequent meetings thereafter to keep it on the agenda. In December 2006, wording for a temporary plaque, approved after consultation with PSAT members and using words from one of our proposed plaques, was placed near the west wall where the construction had begun on the redevelopment.

While the temporary plaque did not tell nearly as much as PSAT members proposed, it was an important and encouraging start. It was the first historical marker anywhere in Canada that acknowledges the *unpaid labour* of psychiatric patients and their "immense" work in maintaining the public asylum system, a practice which was common throughout the country (Moran 2000, 91–95; Dyck and Deighton 2017, 56–57, 66; McKay 2017, 99–116). This collaboration also led to a phone-in service at CAMH, beginning in July 2007, in which a shortened version of the original plaque texts were made available for people to call and listen to, spoken by two psychiatric survivors, Ruth Stackhouse and former Queen Street patient and PSAT co-founder Mel Starkman.[5] Yet, on the road to these plaques, there were cracks along the way.

These different efforts to collaborate have also given way to tensions, nowhere more evident than in a photo exhibit sponsored by CAMH a few months after this phone line tour went into operation. This exhibit included photos by a local photographer who took photos of the wall after he heard that it had writings and drawings on it, likely inscribed by the patients themselves, something which had previously been pointed out on wall tours. The photographer met first with me and then members of PSAT at a meeting in February 2006. PSAT members were tentatively supportive of his project to photographically record the writings by patients on the wall. Members of the archives, however, also expressed concern about someone who was not part of the community appropriating this history for his own purposes. The photographer acknowledged the group's concerns and said he would provide the archives with a copy of his photos for research purposes. Over a year and a half later, this same photographer, who had no further contact with the archives or the psychiatric survivor community, held his photo exhibit about the wall under the auspices of the CAMH Foundation which received proceeds from the sale of his work. The photographer ignored the psychiatric survivor community and his previous commitment to the archives in the process of putting on this exhibit, including when Lucy Costa, a staff member of the CAMH Empowerment Council, worked with PSAT to co-sponsor a "Mad Voices from the Wall" discussion at the gallery holding this exhibit.[6]

---

5   The idea for this phone-in service came from Ed Janiszewski, CAMH Archives volunteer and ally of PSAT, who proposed using the plaque wording developed and endorsed by PSAT for an audio phone tour in spring 2007. This was agreed upon and Ed organized the recording with psychiatric survivors, Ruth Stackhouse and Mel Starkman. This phone line service was put on a CAMH extension in July 2007 and continues to be heard fifteen years later in 2022 at 416-535-8501, ext. 31530.

6   The Empowerment Council and PSAT organized event took place on October 27, 2007 at the exhibiting gallery. It was entitled: "Mad Voices from the Wall: A photo exhibit of patient

Press reports also ignored the long-standing work of the psychiatric survivor community in publicizing and preserving the history of the patient-built wall and instead interpreted the building of the wall by patients as a "therapeutic exercise".[7] The photographer was an active participant in promoting a distorted, white-washed version of history when, in one news story, he is paraphrased as stating, "it was symbolic because the wall provided privacy for those people who were stigmatized for their illness. Now the exhibit and CAMH's decision to keep the structure as a monument during their redevelopment breaks down the barriers of stigma." ("Voices speak for those stigmatized" 2007). The wall is thus a benign structure, even a friend of patients – it does not confine them, it protects their privacy. Moreover, it is the mental health facility which alone is credited for preserving the wall – psychiatric survivors' efforts to preserve the wall are thus of no more consequence to the photographer than historical truths about exploitation and oppression which the wall represents. Perhaps the most distorting report was by the Canadian Broadcasting Company which, in a news story on national television stated that the wall's history had been silent until this 2007 photo exhibit – an astonishing claim after nearly a decade of public history about this wall by mad activists, without whom the history of who built this wall, so widely known by then, would not have been otherwise acknowledged. The Chief Executive Officer of the facility, Paul Garfinkel, stated further in the CBC news story that the wall is "an important symbol for us", claiming a history which psychiatric survivors fought years to have preserved as symbolizing asylum inmates' neglected past first and foremost, something which these reports ignored and co-opted without context or credit (CBC TV 2007).[8] The accounts in the newspapers and television were devoid of historical controversy and told from the points of view of a psychiatrist and a photographer, neither of whom identified as ex-psychiatric patients.

---

writings from the patient built wall", thus emphasizing patients' history in the title of the event in contrast to the photographer's exhibition title which has his name, front and centre, with the patient's history only noted in the fine print.

7   "Not just another brick in the wall", *Toronto Star*, October 23, 2007. To this newspaper's credit, a more historically accurate article was published almost two years later making clear the exploitative nature of the history of these brick walls: Adrian Morrow, "If only the walls of these psychiatric institutions could talk," *Toronto Star*, July 13, 2009. See also: "Psychiatric institutions' walls built by patients: Researcher", *Metro News* [Torstar news service], July 13, 2009, 4.

8   I would like to thank the late Lynne Moss Sharman, Thunder Bay, Ontario, for providing me with a taped copy of this news story soon after it was televised. The words recorded from this report were transcribed by me while listening to this audio-visual tape.

To counter these distortions and to hold the photographer to account, an article was written in the free mass-circulation daily weekly magazine *NOW* by myself, critiquing the exhibit and raising questions about who gets to tell this history and why (Reaume 2007).[9] The photographer was asked to respond in the same issue by the magazine editors. He side-stepped his responsibility, by dishonestly claiming in print that "these people" – members of the Psychiatric Survivor Archives – have "not talked to me" about our concerns which, fortunately, could be disproved by four witnesses and by an email from the photographer himself shortly after our meeting in February 2006.[10] Only after the appearance of this article took him to task, three weeks after the end of this exhibit, did the photographer send by mail a copy of the images he promised to PSAT which was received a month after the exhibit took place.[11]

Three days after the article in *NOW* was published, I took a group of psychiatric survivors on a wall tour and noticed that the temporary plaque publicly acknowledging the patients' labour, which has been in place at this facility for eleven months by then, had been removed; it was there just two weeks earlier when I had given another tour. Official disapproval perhaps of the *NOW* magazine article? Or a coincidence? Unrelated surrounding signage had also been taken down at the same time. I was told the signage was taken down as the construction was nearing completion in that area and the fence was to come down, though the construction fence stayed up for several more months.

---

9   The use of the word "slaved" in the story's subtitle was written by an editor and was not seen by me until publication. I have always opposed comparisons between inmates' labour and slavery whenever someone raises it in discussing this history.

10   The response of photographer, Tom Lackey, and a representative of CAMH, Susan Pigott, are at the bottom of page 20 of the 2007 "Stonewalling survivors" article. At the PSAT meeting of February 18, 2006, attended by Lackey, the following is recorded in the minutes regarding the comments of PSAT member Erick Fabris: "Erick raised issues about appropriation of voice and how psychiatric survivors need to be careful when people come in from outside the community and take over what belongs properly to psychiatric survivors." Erick's concerns were supported by the other members present at this meeting: Lucy Costa, Mel Starkman and myself. Three days later, on February 21, 2006, Lackey acknowledged the concerns that were expressed to him by PSAT members at this meeting in an email which he sent to me in which he wrote: "Thanks for the chance to present my project to the group. The comments and concerns expressed in the discussion afterward were interesting and important for me to hear."

11   The exhibit, called "Voices from the Wall: An exhibition of photographs by Tom Lackey" was held at Lennox Gallery, just north of CAMH from October 25–28, 2007. The *NOW* article appeared on November 15, 2007. Lackey sent a CD and listing of the photos to PSAT from his Toronto address which was received by me at York University for the archives on November 23, 2007.

4   Moving beyond Cracks in the Wall: Proceeding to Plaques,
       2008–2010

Following this episode, there was a lull in consultations for a few months but
by mid-2008, consultation continued between PSAT and CAMH which led to
agreement about a series of nine commemorative plaques to commemorate
patients' labour history on this site. It was agreed that one plaque with mainly
text would be located at the most visible corner of the wall on the northeast
side, describing the history of exploitation and the abilities of patient labourers on this site. It was also agreed that eight additional plaques would be placed
around the rest of the grounds with shorter text than was originally proposed.
Included on each plaque is a large historical image about the social significance of patients' work around the grounds with a link noted at the bottom to
the longer text on the phone extension. This was a compromise from the original PSAT proposal since the first plaque's draft wording in 2005 was to have far
more text than image. However, Susan Piggot of CAMH who proposed these
changes, argued that plaques with large amounts of text, as PSAT was propos-
ing, would have less impact and attraction for passersby, than a brief text on
eight plaques with concise wording, with only one plaque to be primarily text
at the most visible location at Queen and Shaw. Given how quickly people go
by a plaque, being able to grab their attention is crucial. That is why PSAT had
always proposed the plaque with the most overall detail about this history be
located at the corner of Queen and Shaw streets, literally in the shadow of the
east wall built in 1888–89. There is a stoplight here which requires passersby
to pause and thus, hopefully, to notice this historical plaque and the history it
details while waiting for the light to change.

    While there is less historical information on the eight plaques located
around the other parts of the grounds than was first proposed by PSAT, the
information that is on these plaques is direct and to the point about patient
labour in relation to the historical wall so that the message about this history
is immediately clear due to the conciseness of the wording which in every case
notes that patient labourers were not paid or did "free" work for the asylum.
Though reducing the wording on the plaques also reduced historical details
to be contained therein, PSAT ensured that the historical message about the
exploitation of patient labour was *the* overriding theme that brought all of
these plaques together. By making the wording shorter in content, the result
was a directness that was missing from the original longer versions, a change
which increased the chances that people would both read the plaques and get
the message, attracted initially by the large historical images of various people

and places on the grounds on each plaque. The plaque with the most words on it, at Queen and Shaw, has a colourful map of the old asylum grounds to attract people, while superimposed upon it is the location of the eight other plaques around the property. The fact that each plaque notes patients were not paid for their labour was done both to emphasize this point as it relates to each theme described on the plaques, while also ensuring that if a person came upon only one of the plaques at a time since they are scattered around a large urban site, the message of exploitation of labour would be maintained as a unifying theme no matter how many plaques a visitor sees.

There were initially suggestions in discussions with CAMH that this emphasis on unpaid labour on each plaque was redundant, however, I argued, as the PSAT representative, that most people were not likely to see all nine plaques at once, but only come across one or two of them at a time. This increased the need to preserve the centrality of this theme of unpaid patient labour as being crucial for each plaque to ensure that the historical integrity of this message is not lost at any point along the commemorative wall plaques, no matter how many a passerby views. It was also noted that it is essential that the words "exploited labour" appear on the main descriptive plaque at Queen and Shaw describing the historical importance of this legacy for all to read in clear, unequivocal terms, something PSAT insisted upon and to which CAMH agreed. Only by dealing with such unpleasant aspects of history where it happened can we hope to change attitudes and practices for the better, particularly when addressing a group who have been so long marginalized both as workers and citizens in our society. The plaques are meant, therefore, to remember the contributions of previously forgotten people to promote the message that such injustices be learned from and challenged wherever they occur. It is also to ensure that patients' unpaid labour is not whitewashed as "therapeutic" and thus excused as undeserving of compensation, as has been done too often when this past has been interpreted by those who have not lived it.

At PSAT's suggestion, it was agreed in 2008 that the plaques would be installed in 2010 to mark the 150th anniversary of the oldest part of the wall on the south side which was built in 1860. In the meantime, PSAT undertook to raise the approximately $8,000 that was estimated as the cost to produce the wall plaques. Fundraising for the wall plaques began in earnest in the spring of 2009 with the commencement of wall tours at the end of which a flyer was handed out from PSAT outlining the purpose of the plaques, their estimated cost and asking for donations which, for most of the time until near the very end of the fundraising effort, the archives was not able to offer a tax receipt due to our not having a charitable number.[12] People were generous in donating on the spot and, more often, sending cheques to PSAT's mailing address. Organisations also made generous donations, including the CAMH Friends of the Archives and CAMH as well. These fundraising efforts culminated on April 21, 2010 with a "Words on the Wall" event held at the nearby nineteenth-century Gladstone Hotel. Initiated and organized by PSAT member Andrea White along with Chris Reed of This Is Not a Reading Series, over forty local artists created artistically rendered bricks which were auctioned at a public event near the historical site with bricks donated by CAMH, many from a 1970s hospital patio that was being dismantled. Some of the bricks were irreverent, as with a Teddy Bear brick for "prescription hugs" to more sombre in tone, with another brick imprisoned behind bars with a woman's dress imprinted on it representing gender discrimination in mad people's history. Other creatively used bricks included one which an artist had encased entirely in glass on every side, while another one was surrounded by a tree bark whilst still another one had been literally ground down into a dust in a square box in which people were invited to rearrange the remains any way they chose to do so. Over $2,300 was raised at this event with over one hundred people in attendance, pushing the total amount to over the $8,000 figure estimated as needed to pay for the plaques. In doing so, this event gave the wider community "ownership" and literal investment in commemorating mad people's labour history in a way that carried forward the creativity of the past into the present, though without the exploitation of those whom these plaques remember.[13]

In July 2010, at the PSAT Annual General Meeting, an unveiling date was proposed of September 25th for the wall plaques which was agreed upon by CAMH and the wall plaque makers in Quebec, Systeme Huntingdon, who had been contracted to supply the final product. Due to the tight timelines in wanting to meet this schedule, a great deal of pressure was felt on all sides

---

12   Until April 2010, all donors who gave money to PSAT for the wall plaques were not able to receive a tax receipt due to the archives not having charitable status. In April 2010, Heritage Toronto, the local municipal historical preservation association, kindly allowed donors for the wall plaques to use their tax receipt number for this purpose which was advertised by PSAT during the final stages of fundraising.

13   From fall 2008, when the first fundraising was started, though most money was raised beginning from spring 2009, PSAT raised $8,113.02 (of which $7,058.02 was raised without benefit of a tax receipt for donors; $1055 was able to be provided with a tax receipt, as is explained in the preceding note). The total cost of the plaques was less than estimated at $6,676.04. CAMH helped to defray this cost by paying for the actual installation on site. This left $1,436.98 remaining in the PSAT credit union account from the wall plaques' fundraising campaign.

as the plaques were delayed in getting to the site until literally the day before their widely advertised launch; the pedestals upon which the plaques are mounted had arrived a couple of days before and were placed in the ground while the plaques arrived on September 24.[14] Originally, the plan had been to place the plaques directly on the walls, except for the first descriptive plaque at the corner of Queen and Shaw which was always agreed should be on a pedestal for better positioning at this corner. However, after further consideration, including consultation with Heritage Toronto who expressed concerns about placing plaques on the east wall in particular due to the need for further conservation work, it was decided that all nine plaques would go on pedestals directly in front of, or very close to, the wall at designated spots. In each case, the location of the plaque was based on where the theme of each individual plaque matched the historical location: women's work, including domestic toil, laundry and sewing; men's work including construction, maintenance and agricultural labour; as well as related themes such as where bodies of patients were prepared for burial atop a former barn. Thanks to the dedicated work of CAMH staff members and contract staff who ensured the deadline was met, all nine plaques were installed one day before the unveiling ceremony; fortunately, the weather cooperated in allowing the cement to dry in time.

This literally last-minute activity allowed the unveiling to proceed on Saturday, September 25, 2010, after a decade of talking about it and five years after drafting the first written proposals for the plaques, followed by various revisions. Before the final version of the plaques were sent to the plaque makers, CAMH Archivist John Court, a strong supporter of PSAT's preservation efforts from the beginning, selected a number of historical images from the CAMH Archives related to the various themes on each plaque and presented them to the wider group for feedback. CAMH Archives board member Ed Janiszewski brought forward an 1863 plan of the asylum grounds from the provincial archives which is on the main descriptive plaque on which the location of the eight other plaques are noted and I provided images of two patients, one male and one female, with permission of the Archives of Ontario where these photos were found in patient files. With this collective effort of the above-mentioned participants, as well as Mel Starkman of PSAT and CAMH staff, it was agreed on the best images to use, which were shown to other members of the organizing parties in PSAT and CAMH. In addition to

---

14   A few days before the plaques arrived, John Court, CAMH Archivist, myself and construction work staff members went around the CAMH property to specify exactly where each plaque would be located which followed the route of the wall tours since 2000.

the 1863 map of the old asylum grounds, plaque images also include historical images of the old north wall which no longer exists right behind two daughters of a groundskeeper; the nurses' residence where woman patients worked as domestic servants; photos of exteriors of long since demolished ninteteenth-century buildings where patients lived, worked and died; an interior image of a workshop with a staff carpenter where patients worked and which is one of two small nineteenth-century patient built buildings that still exist alongside the walls; a photo of agricultural labourers taken in the 1920s at the nearby Mimico Asylum three miles west of Queen Street to represent male patient field workers; and of particular importance, two images of patients who lived and worked on these grounds: a photo of Audrey B. taken in 1937 located on a plaque which mentions that she worked in the asylum sewing room for at least thirty years; and a photo of Jim P. walking several dogs on the grounds in 1927 who toiled in the nearby workshop. Together, Audrey and Jim are reminders of the thousands of women and men patients whose unpaid work at long last has the permanent public recognition that the patient-built walls represent and are described on these plaques for all to see. That recognition was witnessed at the unveiling on September 25, 2010 by people who attended the event and continues every time someone goes by any one of these plaques and reads or hears about the work psychiatric patients did on these grounds (Morriss 2010; Reaume 2010).

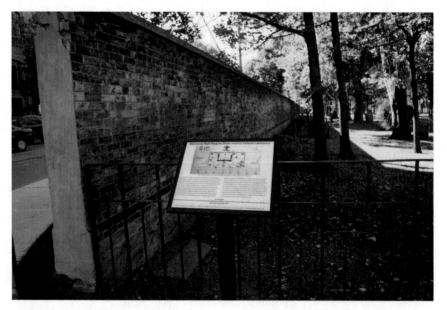

FIGURE 6.3A   Geoffrey Reaume, main interpretative plaque near 1888–89 east wall

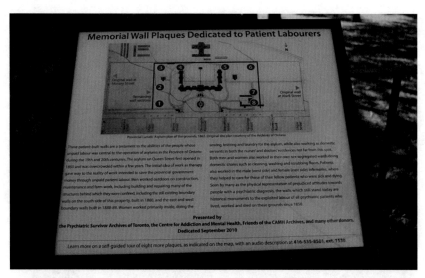

FIGURE 6.3B   PSAT & CAMH Archives, memorial wall plaques dedicated to patient labouers

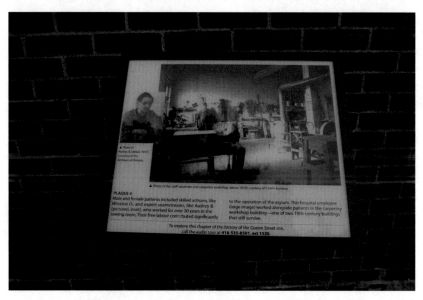

FIGURE 6.4   Geoffrey Reaume, Audrey B and female patients' labour in the sewing room &
laundry

A year after the unveiling of these plaques, in October 2011, Heritage
Toronto awarded the Psychiatric Survivor Archives its annual "Community
Heritage Award" stating in their citation: "The jury felt this group accom-
plished a lot with very little, using creative ways to fundraise and make their

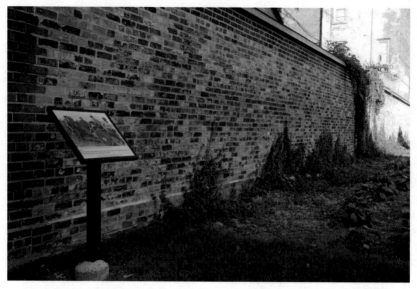

FIGURE 6.5   Geoffrey Reaume, agricultural labourers near former site of barnyard and
              gate along west wall

cause known. The jury also commended the work of the Psychiatric Survivor Archives in recognizing the significant contributions that a marginalized
community has made to the City's fabric, shedding light on a little-known
dimension of Toronto's history." ("Shedding light ..." 2011).

5   Academic Critiques of These Efforts: Reaction and Revision

Of course, the installation of the plaques is not the end of reinterpreting this
wall's history. There have been scholarly reactions which oppose these efforts
to critically interpret mad people's history in public commemorations. A year
after the plaques were installed, two historians, Nathan Flis and David Wright,
wrote that these commemoration efforts are a "subtle new form of anti-
psychiatry, where motifs borrowed from memorialisations of the Holocaust,
the First World War, and American slavery are adapted to the political aspirations of 'psychiatric survivors' organizations. Aided by a sympathetic press [...]
[and] senior figures of the psychiatric establishment who [...] have paradoxically embraced problematic narratives of their own profession's past." (Flis and
Wright 2011, 102).[15] They further state that references to unpaid labour at the

---

15   In their 2011 article, Flis and Wright state that the organizing group is called the "Psychiatric
      Survivors Association of Toronto" when the correct name during its entire existence was

nineteenth-century Toronto Asylum are "an allusion to slave labour – as in the war-time camps during World War II or in the Communist China labour colonies [which] drives home the point of exploitation as a central theme in the history of the mental hospital." (Flis and Wright 2011, 108–109). Flis and Wright make no attempt in their article to define what they mean by "anti-psychiatry" and how it is directly comparable to commemorative efforts on the Toronto Asylum patient-built wall. Using a loaded and vague term like "anti-psychiatry" to critique commemorative efforts of mad people's history is a way of trying to marginalize and counter such efforts. The supposed "allusions" referring to historical motifs, such as the Holocaust and American slavery have never been part of the promotion or interpretation of unpaid patients' labour history by myself or PSAT as an organization. Indeed, I am on record as opposing such comparisons even before the archives came into existence as is stated in an article published in the *Canadian Bulletin of Medical History* in 2000. Referring to the analogy that has been invoked in comparing crimes in Nazi Germany with psychiatric practices in contemporary North America, I wrote, in part: "We should be able to make our criticisms of whoever it is who is being criticized on its own merits (or demerits) without resorting to this massively overused reference to one of history's most horrific periods." (Reaume 2000b, note 47, 120–121).

The claims of being "Aided by a sympathetic press" are also vastly overstated – while the *Toronto Star* did publish two articles six years apart (2003 and 2009) on efforts to preserve this wall's history, overall, the mainstream print, electronic and radio media did not cover these efforts (Sorensen 2003; Morrow 2009). There was no mainstream media coverage of the unveiling of the wall plaques in 2010 or of the fundraising efforts in the months prior to this and the media citations they use to 'prove' this point are unconnected to

---

the "The Psychiatric Survivor Archives of Toronto." They also claim that I was its Director which is also not true as no such position ever existed in this organization. Instead, I was elected Chairperson (2007–12) and I was one of four co-founders of PSAT which started in 2001 (the three other co-founders being Janet Bruch, Mel Starkman and Don Weitz). The two authors make a number of other mistakes about the history of the archives in their article besides not getting its name right, including claiming that Gail Hornstein, a professor of psychology from Massachusetts is a member of PSAT which is totally false (I met her once, the year before PSAT was founded, at a medical history conference in Bethesda, Maryland in 2000; we exchanged two or three emails afterwards). Flis and Wright also write that the archives have been in existence "over the last two decades" which, at the time their article was published is one decade too many, and that during my wall tours of the patient built walls, I refer to "the wooden spiral staircase that originally led up to the front/central water tower" which is also not accurate as I seldom ever mentioned this object which could not be seen on the wall tour in any case: Flis and Wright (2011), all citations above from page 109.

the wall plaques' campaign and do not support their arguments. Critics of the term "exploitation" in regard to unpaid asylum patient labour, such as Flis and Wright, should develop criticism of this argument based on its own merits instead of resorting to false "allusions" which have never been made by this historian in the first place. To do otherwise constructs a false historiography based on their own illusory allusions. It is also an attempt to downplay and excuse the historical economic exploitation of mad and disabled peoples' labour in institutions as a form of "therapy" even though historical research has shown that unpaid patients' work was used as a source of cheap labour (Beckwith 2016; Rose 2017). There were some senior administrative staff at the current Centre for Addiction and Mental Health who did assist these efforts – and this is a crucial point which troubles Flis and Wright but for the wrong reasons.

In their article, Flis and Wright note that in our efforts to preserve the patient-built walls, there was an "unusual alliance between PSAT and the psychiatric elite of CAMH." (Flis and Wright 2011, 109). Nowhere in their article do the authors note the central reason for this "unusual alliance": the patient-built boundary walls are on CAMH property and any effort to preserve and publicly commemorate patients' labour which these walls represent must involve the facility which is directly responsible for their continued existence and long-term maintenance. PSAT would not have been able to get anywhere in our efforts if we did not deal with CAMH directly in this historical work since the patient-built walls are on their property. This "alliance" can only be depicted as "unusual" if this essential piece of history is ignored. It would be "unusual" for any group seeking to preserve and interpret an aspect of history anywhere to not work with the owners of a property that is the focus of such efforts. The archives had to work with the administration there to preserve the wall and get permanent plaques installed, otherwise its preservation and public interpretation would have been, quite literally, out of our hands. Yes, this history can be and has been co-opted by the psychiatric establishment for their own ends. Such co-option deserves critical scrutiny. There also needs to be an acknowledgement that when we move our historical scholarship beyond the ivory tower, the benefits of making critical interpretations of mad people's history more accessible to the wider community are far greater than the risks. Indeed, a literally concrete example of such benefits can be found in an article written nearly a decade after the plaques were installed. In 2019, a person completely unknown to this author wrote an article in a construction trade newsletter about preservation work being done on the east wall at that time. After describing the significance of the patient-built wall's history and the type of preservation work being undertaken, Peter Kenter ends his article with a direct quote from the last sentence on the main plaque by the east wall being a monument "to the exploited labour" of psychiatric patients, as can be found in the image of this plaque included in this chapter. He then concludes with his own words: "The current restoration work will ensure that this history is never forgotten." (Kenter 2019, 3).

6   Conclusion

What would happen to this history if mad activists did not work collaboratively on a particular heritage project owned by the psychiatric establishment? It would have been a mistake of huge proportions since that would have precluded any advocacy role in both preserving and publicly interpreting our past. Certainly, the word "exploitation" having been included on the main descriptive plaque on the grounds of the former Toronto Asylum, and ensuring that patients' unpaid or "free" labour is mentioned on all of the remaining plaques only happened because members of the Psychiatric Survivor Archives had been involved in this process from beginning until end. Engaging this past as a public historian is crucial in fighting prejudices in the present by addressing contemporary social justice struggles around social exclusion and exploitation which these old walls represent. Otherwise, if these walls were to be publicly interpreted at all, it would have been as the history of an architect and doctors. Activist efforts to preserve the nineteenth-century Toronto Asylum patient built boundary walls were based upon respecting psychiatric patients' unpaid work that public interpretations have traditionally ignored. Indeed, if there is a "grave injustice" to which Flis and Wright refer, it is that it has taken so long to get this history of exploitation publicly acknowledged or even seriously addressed by historians. Above all, these efforts are inspired by the people who lived this history and a desire to make mad people's history accessible and relevant to the wider community to whom it belongs.

Dedication

This article is dedicated to the memory of Graeme Bacque (1958–2021), a long-time member and supporter of the Psychiatric Survivor Archives of Toronto, among many other social justice organisations. Graeme helped with the memorial plaques campaign described in this chapter in countless ways over many years.

References

Annual Report of the Inspector of Asylums, Prisons and Public Charities. 1890.

Beckwith, Ruthie-Marie. 2016. *Disability Servitude: From Peonage to Poverty*. New York: Palgrave Macmillan US.

CBC TV National News. 2007. October 25.

City of Toronto By-Law No. 1997-0085. 1996. Schedule "B", Heritage Property Report, Recording Date, September 1996.

Court, John. 2000. "From 999 to 1001 Queen Street: A Consistently Vital Resource." In *The Provincial Asylum in Toronto: Reflections on Social and Architectural History*, edited by Edna Hudson, 183–198. Toronto: Toronto Region Architectural Conservancy.

Dyck, Erika, and Alex Deighton. 2017. *Managing Madness: Weyburn Mental Hospital and the Transformation of Psychiatric Care in Canada*. Winnipeg: University of Manitoba Press.

Flis, Nathan, and David Wright. 2011. "'A Grave Injustice': The Mental Hospital and Shifting Sites of Memory." In *Exhibiting Madness in Museums: Remembering Psychiatry through Collections and Display*, edited by Catherine Coleborne and Dolly MacKinnon, 101–115. London: Routledge.

Kenter, Peter. 2019. "Restoration of CAMH walls preserves important chapter of patient history." *Daily Commercial News by Construct Connect*, August 6, 3.

McKay, Kathryn. 2016. "From Blasting Powder to Tomato Pickles: Patient Work at the Provincial Mental Hospitals in British Columbia, Canada, c. 1885–1920." In *Work, Psychiatry and Society, c. 1750–2015*, edited by Waltraud Ernst, 99–116. Manchester: Manchester University Press.

Moran, James E. 2000. *Committed to the State Asylum: Insanity and Society in Nineteenth-Century Quebec and Ontario*. Montreal & Kingston: McGill-Queen's University Press.

Morriss, Shirley. 2010. "Recovering and Celebrating Our Past." *Friends of the Archives Newsletter* [CAMH] 18, no. 2 (October).

Morrow, Adrian. 2009. "If Only the Walls of these Psychiatric Institutions Could Talk." *Toronto Star*, July 13.

"Not Just another Brick in the Wall." 2007. *Toronto Star*, October 23.

"Psychiatric Institutions' Walls Built by Patients: Researcher." 2009. *Metro News* [Torstar news service], July 13.

Punzi, Elisabeth. 2019. "Ghost Walks or Thoughtful Remembrance: How should the heritage of psychiatry be approached?" *The Journal of Critical Psychology, Counselling and Psychotherapy* 19, no. 4 (December): 242–251.

Reaume, Geoffrey. 2000a. *Remembrance of Patients Past: Patient Life at the Toronto Hospital for the Insane*. Toronto: Oxford University Press.

Reaume, Geoffrey. 2000b. "Portraits of People with Mental Disorders in English Canadian History." *Canadian Bulletin of Medical History* 17, no. 1&2: 93–125.

Reaume, Geoffrey. 2006. "Patients at Work: Insane Asylum Inmate Labour in Ontario, 1841–1900." In *Mental Health and Canadian Society: Historical Perspectives*, edited by James Moran and David Wright, 69–96. Montreal/Kingston: McGill-Queen's University Press.

Reaume, Geoffrey. 2007. "Stonewalling survivors: Who gets to tell the history of patients who slaved for the Toronto Asylum wall?" *NOW* [weekly magazine, Toronto], November 15–21: 20–21.

Reaume, Geoffrey. 2010. "These walls are the last remaining witnesses ..." *Voices: Newsletter of the Psychiatric Survivor Archives*, Toronto, 1, no. 3 (November): 1–3, 6.

Reaume, Geoffrey. 2010–2011. "Psychiatric Patient Built Wall Tours at the Centre for Addiction and Mental Health (CAMH), Toronto, 2000–2010." *Left History* 15, no. 1 (Fall/Winter): 127–146.

Reaume, Geoffrey. 2017. "From the Perspectives of Mad People." In *The Routledge History of Madness and Mental Health*, edited by Greg Eghigian, 277–296. London: Routledge.

Rose, Sarah F. 2017. *No Right to be Idle: The Invention of Disability, 1840s-1930s*. Chapel Hill: University of North Carolina Press.

"Shedding Light on a Little-Known Dimension of Toronto's History." 2011. *Voices: Newsletter of the Psychiatric Survivor Archives*, Toronto 2, no. 3 (October): 3.

Sorensen, Chris. 2003. "Future of Shaw Street Wall in Doubt." *Toronto Star*, February 13.

"Voices Speak for Those Stigmatized by Illness." 2007. *24 Hours*, October 24.

Yellow Bird, Pemina. 2004. "Wild Indians: Native Perspectives on the Hiawatha Asylum for Insane Indians." Open access at: dsmc.info/pdf/canton.pdf.

CHAPTER 7

Street Names and the Narration of Madness in a Post-Asylum Landscape

Cecilia Rodéhn

Abstract

The aim of this article is to discuss street naming at Ulleråker, a former psychiatric hospital located in the town Uppsala in southeastern Sweden. Specifically, the article explores streets named after Gustaf Fröding's poems: what kinds of stories are narrated in the urban landscape when Fröding's poems are used as inspiration for street names? Fröding (1860–1911) is a well-known Swedish writer and poet who was an inmate at Ulleråker. Furthermore, the article explores the cultural heritage this produces in the post-asylum landscape. The street-naming process and the street names are subjected to a mad reading, and the article adopts theories and methodologies from Critical Heritage Studies, Human Geography, and Mad Studies. I argue that the street naming builds on sanist discourses that further gendered and classed stereotypes of people diagnosed with mental distress. These discourses are then subverted, and the article shows how the street names narrate and materialize different kinds of experiences of madness in the post-asylum landscape.

Keywords

Gustaf Fröding – mad leakage – mad reading – street naming – Ulleråker – post-asylum landscape

1 Introduction

In 2016, the local government decided that some streets in the Ulleråker post-asylum landscape should be named after the famous Swedish poet Gustaf Fröding and his poems. Founded in 1811, Ulleråker, located in the town Uppsala in Southeast Sweden, has a more than two-hundred-year-old history as a psychiatric hospital area. The hospital was deinstitutionalized in 1988 and is an example of a typical Swedish post-asylum landscape. Ebba Högström explains

© KONINKLIJKE BRILL BV, LEIDEN, 2025 | DOI:10.1163/9789004519848_009

that Swedish post-asylum landscapes can be considered as "an effect of the overall restructuring of social welfare services and as the result of processes of rationalisation, reductions in public funding and a shift from the previously dominant model of public supply to mixed public–private solutions" (2018, 317). Moreover, a post-asylum landscape is a new kind of spatialisation of hospital areas, where they are subject to urban development and re-envisioned as business areas, school campuses, prisons, and residential areas (Moon, Kearns, and Joseph 2015). From the late 1980s, Ulleråker has been transformed from hospital grounds into a residential area and school campuses. The land is currently subject to large-scale urban development, which began in 2014. A central part of the urban development of Swedish post-asylum landscapes is the introduction of new street names. At Ulleråker, new street names were first introduced during the 1990s, commemorating one nurse and five attending physicians who had worked at the hospital. Later, during the urban development process starting in 2014, it was decided, as mentioned above, that new streets should be named after the poet Gustaf Fröding and his poems (Stadsbyggnadsförvaltningen 2016).

Gustaf Fröding is one of Sweden's best-known and cherished poets. He was born on August 22, 1860, in the county of Värmland in southwestern Sweden. Fröding arrived in Uppsala as a student, and he lived there, as well as in Stockholm, with his sisters. He debuted with a collection of poems named *Guitar and Concertina* (*Guitarr och dragharmonika*) in 1891, which was followed in 1894 by *New Poems* (*Nya dikter*). In 1896, *Splashes and Patches* (Stänk och flikar) was published followed by *Tall Tales and Adventures* (*Räggler å paschaser*) in 1895, *Old and New* (*Nytt och gammalt*) in 1897 and *Splashes of the Grail* (*Gralstänk*) in 1898. In private, the author suffered from mental ill-health, and Fröding was treated at many different care facilities in Europe. On December 28, 1898, he was admitted to Uppsala Hospital at Ulleråker, where he was diagnosed with "Insania degenerativa", meaning "inherited mental illness". Fröding remained in care until March 21, 1905, when he was released to his sisters and cared for by a private nurse in his home in Stockholm. Fröding died February 8, 1911 (Jonsson 2002, 11). His work is part of the Swedish literary canon, and his life and work continue to inspire musicians, filmmakers, and playwrights.

The aim of this article is to examine what histories are narrated in the urban landscape when Fröding's poems are used as inspiration for street names. Furthermore, the article explores what kind of cultural heritage this produces in Ulleråker's post-asylum landscape. In this exploration, the article contributes to the ongoing discussion of name-giving at psychiatric hospital areas. In this field of study, scholars have explored place names, suggesting that post-asylum landscapes are often subject to radical name changes during urban development (Moon, Kearns, and Joseph 2015, 73, 84–87, 122–126, 162). Robin Kearns, Alun Joseph and Graham Moon write that this is because a stigma is often attached to former psychiatric hospital sites due to their association with the care of people diagnosed with "mental illness" (Kearns, Joseph, and Moon 2012, 180). They conclude that renaming former psychiatric hospital areas often becomes a strategy and a tool by urban developers and politicians to cleanse the place of negative associations. New names function as a way to create a symbolic break with the past in the process of creating attractive residential areas (Moon, Kearns, and Joseph 2015, 84–87, 122–126, 162). Although place names are discussed, street naming and street names have not been subject to analysis; the present article contributes in this regard.

Furthermore, the present article contributes to the discussion by examining the kinds of histories that are narrated when introducing new street names into an urban area (e.g. Azaryahu 1996, 2012; Gill 2005; Ryan, Foote, and Azaryahu 2016). This body of work predominantly examines processes of naming streets in relation to major political transitions in various countries (e.g. Gill 2005; Palonen 2008; Duminy 2017; Shoval 2013; Light and Young 2014; Wanjiru and Matsubara 2017). Though an important focus, the interest has sidelined research into more mundane street naming processes, and, consequently, small-scale political processes are often overlooked. The present study contributes in this regard by focusing on political decisions on local levels. Furthermore, in building on research that explores how histories are narrated and commemorated in the urban landscape (Azaryahu 1996; 2012; Light 2004; Palonen 2008), research that explores how some pasts are forgotten in order to create new presents and futures (Gill 2005, 492), as well as research exploring the kinds of claims being made when previously subjugated groups' stories are told (Azaryahu 1996; Azaryahu 2012; Winjiru and Mtsubara 2017; Duminy 2017), this article seeks to continue the discussion on how marginalized groups are commemorated by focusing on a group that has not previously been discussed in this context: people diagnosed with "mental illness".

2   Points of Departure

Methodologically and theoretically, this article is located at the intersection of Critical Heritage Studies, Human Geography and Mad Studies. Within Human Geography Maoz Azaryahu suggests that street names narrate the officially sanctioned history and heritage of an area (1996; 2012). Yet, it is acknowledged that street names are not narrative in and of themselves but that they have a narrative (Ryan, Foote, and Azaryahu 2016, 158–159). Further, Marie-Laure

Ryan, Kenneth Foote and Maoz Azaryahu write that for something to be a narrative it needs a sequel structure, a story line, or a complete narrative. They suggest that street names lack this. However, having a narrative implies that street names are a medium through which narratives are realized (Ryan, Foote, and Azaryahu 2016, 158–159). They hold that street names have the capacity to tell old and/or new stories in the urban landscape, and street names are also in and of themselves materializations of stories (Ryan, Foote, and Azaryahu 2016, 139–141, 153). Street names are thus "participants in the ongoing cultural production of a shared past" (Azaryahu 1996, 312). Seen in this light, street naming is a place where Ulleråker's cultural heritage is suggested, negotiated and realized.

To explore this, I have systematically collected and analysed material related to the name-giving process at Ulleråker, collected from Uppsala municipality archives (*Uppsala kommunarkiv*) as well as the Uppsala town's archive (*Uppsala stadsarkiv*). This material includes minutes from meetings, from groups such as the "name-giving board" (*namngivningsnämnden*), the municipality's civic dialogue regarding future names, and official statements made by Uppsala municipality and the name-giving board. I combine this material with my personal communication with a municipality official, who has been made anonymous, and their gender also has been concealed using the pronoun they/their. I further combine this with newspaper articles where municipal officials are interviewed. I consider the material as articulations – representations or meaning-making practices constituted by discourses. Thus, street names can be considered as discursive products as well as sites of memory where power, remembrance, language, and space are conflated (Azaryahu 2012, 388). In keeping with research in Critical Heritage Studies and Human Geography, street naming can be considered a cultural practice and an active performative process, where the past is used in order to create meaning; it is a process of creating cultural heritage (Azaryahu 1996; Azaryahu 2012; Smith 2006, 47). The idea that street names are discursive products (Azaryahu 2012, 388) is central in the discussion of street naming as a cultural heritage process because '[t]he discursive construction of heritage is itself part of the cultural and social processes that are heritage' (Smith 2006, 13).

In order to further examine the discursive constructs of Ulleråker's cultural heritage in terms of street names, I turn to *mad reading*. This is an approach that seeks to make visible how people with mental distress are depicted in different kinds of texts (Wolframe 2014). More specifically, it seeks to examine the "discursive conditions of madness' emergence" with the aim to illuminate expressions of sanism (Wolframe 2014, III, 2, 12, 237). *Madness* is defined as a cultural approach to medicalized experiences and considered a general term for different phenomena indicating distress of some kind in an individual (LeFrançois, Menzies, and Reaume 2013, 337). The word has been reclaimed for liberatory purposes. It signifies a resistance to psychiatry and creates a possibility to view madness more favourably (LeFrançois, Menzies, and Reaume 2013, 337). *Sanism* is a term that describes discrimination against people diagnosed with "mental illness and neuropsychiatric variation", and it includes someone that is seen as having different social behaviour than the perceived norm (LeFrançois, Menzies, and Reaume 2013, 337). A mad reading is what PhebeAnn Wolframe (2014, 143) calls a *maddening*, a term akin to *cripping* that entails exposing the ways in which ableism "get[s] naturalized and the ways that bodies, minds, and impairments that should be at the absolute center of a space or issue or discussion get purged from that space or issue or discussion" (McRuer 2019, 135). Conducting a mad reading further suggests exploring how sanism intersects with other oppressive ideologies such as sexism, racism, classism, ageism, ableism, and transphobia (Wolframe 2014, 12).

In this text, I use mad reading in two ways. First, I adopt mad reading in order to explore how discourses of sanism manifest during the street-naming process with the purpose of exposing how people experiencing madness are othered in cultural heritage processes. Second, I explore how madness can become central in narratives, specifically in the construction of Ulleråker's cultural heritage. A mad reading of street names works with the tension between what is visible/invisible in cultural productions, where the invisible is considered just as important as the visible for understanding representations of madness (Rodéhn 2022). Mad reading seen in this light suggests that street naming that at first appears as sanist may have cracks where madness seeps out; there are, in other words, *mad leakages* (see Rodéhn 2022). Focusing on mad leakages when analysing street names entails reading beyond the visible and seeking out new contexts and connections (Rodéhn 2022). To explore these leakages, I analyse the street names in connection with Fröding's poems used to name the streets as well as Gustaf Fröding's life and his experiences of madness, mental care and hospitalization. I also read the poems in relation to medical and social discourses at the time when they were produced. In doing so, I offer a narrative that centres on the experience of madness. A mad reading can be considered a performance; it is an active undertaking where the researcher searches for different meanings beyond what is considered the "right" or officially sanctioned version of, in this case, a street name. It is also a situation where the researcher actively contributes to creating and mediating these new meanings. Mad reading in this way is not only what Wolframe (2014, 143) calls a *maddening*; it is also a re-centring of the analysis so that those that have been excluded, and their experiences, are not just included in cultural narratives but become, and continue to be, the center of cultural heritage.

In the text that follows, I first explain the name-giving process at Ulleråker. Next, I turn to discuss sanist discourses in the name-giving process and what consequences they have for the cultural heritage at Ulleråker. I then turn to highlighting mad leakages and showing how the street names narrate Fröding's experiences of madness and his critique of social norms and medical discourses.

3   Naming Streets

In Sweden, deciding on and implementing street names is an administrative process (Lantmäteriet 2016). Street names are thus produced in a particular political context (Light and Young 2014, 670), and they are instrumental in validating the ruling socio-political order's view of themselves and of the place (Azaryahu 1996, 312; Gill 2005). In Uppsala Municipality, street naming is carried out by municipal officials and a board for name-giving.

It is common in Sweden that streets are named after the history of the area where they exist (Lantmäteriet 2016). An official at Uppsala Municipality explained this process to the local newspaper: "We look at the area and what existed there previously but also what exists around it" (Winberg 2018, my translation). They added, "I spend quite a lot of time looking at maps" in order to study structures that may be historically significant, because names "have to do with our immaterial cultural heritage and our identity" (Sandow 2016, my translation). In order to better understand the history of the place, the municipal official also held meetings with local museums and heritage officials (Municipal official 2018). When doing research about Ulleråker, the municipal official stated that the poet Gustaf Fröding appeared as a suitable theme for some of the street names (Sandow 2016). They suggested that he "could be seen as symbol for all the tales that have been told about the area" (Sandow 2016, my translation).

Fröding and his poems can also be seen in the civic dialogue organized by the municipality. The civic dialogue was arranged as a meeting where citizens could propose names for streets. The process resulted in 412 suggestions. Among the suggestions were names of doctors, psychologists, researchers and nurses. Suggestions also included different professions and names related to medicine. There were additional names associated with nature and wildlife at Ulleråker, as well as names alluding to the area's diverse history (Namngivningsnämnden 2016). The minutes from the name giving board meeting read that "after the civic dialogue, hosted by the name-giving board, concerning suggestions for name to Ulleråker, over 400 names have been received, several alluding to Gustaf Fröding" (Namngivningsnämndens arbetsutskott 2016, my translation). In actuality, Fröding and his poems were mentioned 23 times. This can be compared to names alluding to the natural environment at Ulleråker, which were mentioned 123 times, and names associated to various states of mind, which were mentioned 83 times (see Namngivningsnämnden 2016). Nevertheless, it was decided that literary references should be a category of names for the streets (Stadsbyggnadsförvaltningen 2016). A few months later, the minutes from the name-giving board meeting state that "the category of names for the area are suggested to be Gustaf Fröding and literary references. The proposed names allude to Gustaf Fröding's poems" (Namngivningsnämndens arbetsutskott 2016, my translation). Eventually, the following names were decided on: Bergtrollsvägen (Mountain Troll Street), Diktens väg (The Poem's Street), Fylgiavägen (Fylgia Street), Levnadsfärden (The Journey of Life), Morgondrömsvägen (Morning Dream Street), Poetens väg (The Poet's Street) and Titaniavägen (Titania Street). Before the decision was made, the street names were displayed in public for consideration, and no objections were made. The names will be implemented after the detailed developing plan is put into practice in the years to come.

4   Gustaf Fröding in the Construction of Ulleråker's Heritage

The claim that Fröding "could be seen as a symbol for all the tales that have been told about the area" (Sandow 2016, my translation), is problematic. Fröding's literary work cannot be made into a universal symbol for all patients' experiences at Ulleråker since he was far from an ordinary patient at the hospital. He was a poet, a celebrity, and his work is part of the Swedish literary canon. At the time of Fröding's hospitalization, it was also well known that he was a patient at Ulleråker. It was mentioned in newspapers, and he was photographed in his hospital bed by a known photographer, Johan Morén. The image was later used by the artist Richard Bergh for his famous painting of the poet from 1909. As a celebrity patient, Fröding has come to occupy a role in the doing of Ulleråker's cultural heritage, and this extends beyond street names.

For instance, the poet is mentioned in the explanation for why Uppsala is of national interest (riksintresse). *National interest* is a concept used by the Swedish National Heritage Board to explain how certain cultural milieus reflect the country's history. It is stated that Uppsala's built environment reflects Sweden's centralised power, the church and the university's history from the

Middle Ages until today (Beckman-Thoor and Holmbäck 2014). Ulleråker is connected to this history, and the hospital is seen as "connected to well-known historical individuals such as the poet Gustaf Fröding [...]" (Beckman-Thoor and Holmbäck 2014, 17, my translation). Fröding not only appears in the description of Uppsala's *national interest*; he also permeates the entire urban development project at Ulleråker, and the poet is used in the marketing of the area. For instance, Uppsala Municipality's homepage states;

> Ulleråker's milieu is charged with stories of those who have lived and worked there, some more colorful than others. [...] [This] can be seen in several patients at Ulleråker, among them the poet Gustaf Fröding (Uppsala kommun 2019, my translation).

Moreover, during the urban development of Ulleråker, Uppsala Municipality has invested in the creative. They have sponsored studios and scholarships for artists, backed art installations in the post-asylum landscape, and opened areas for local entrepreneurs (see Mårdh in this book, pp. 165). This is very much part of a larger neoliberal idea of creating space for the creative class in the urban landscape, and it operates as a means of gentrifying areas. The image of Fröding as a creative patient functions to link creative people of the past and of the present.

Nevertheless, the focus on creativity foregrounds a set of sanist and gendered ideologies and practices that work as a form of "strategic forgetting", a concept that Moon, Kearns, and Joseph explain as a process when a segment of history is deliberately forgotten in order to rebrand the former psychiatric hospital areas (Moon, Kearns, and Joseph 2015, 73, 84–87, 122–126, 162). Building on their writing, I suggest that the focus on creativity, as articulated in the examined material, draws attention to what is considered positive with mental distress and directs attention away from suffering and any uncomfortable feelings connected to madness. As such, it is an effective way to acknowledge and use the past while, at the same time, materializing a more pleasant future.

In terms of Ulleråker, this can be further seen in that no streets are named after Fröding. The only street that alludes to him as a person is Poetens väg (The Poet's Street), perhaps because Frödingsgatan (Fröding's Street) already exists elsewhere in Uppsala. Looking only to the names – Bergtrollsvägen (Mountain Troll Street), Diktens väg (The Poem's Street), Fylgiavägen (Fylgia Street), Levnadsfärden (The Journey of Life), Morgondrömsvägen (Morning Dream Street), Poetens väg (The Poet's Street) and Titaniavägen (Titania Street) – they are at first glance only fanciful names. For those citizens who can make the connection, they are at best reminders of Fröding's literary worlds that incorporate depictions of mythological beings and green lush forests. For some the names may play on a cherished and long-gone Romantic landscape. Titaniavägen, a street named after the poem "Titania", perhaps exemplifies this most clearly. Titania is the queen of elves in Shakespeare's *A Midsummer Night's Dream*, and in the poem, the speaker asks,

> Who *is* this, who's holding her wind-light ball
> at this hour of midnight in moon-silver hall?
>
> FRÖDING 1997 [1891], 61, 2nd stanza, lines 5–6, emphasis in original

In the poem, Fröding depicts the sounds of fiddles whining, sighs between trees, and a full moon floating in a dark forest where elves "in silky gauze dresses" dance (1997 [1891], 61, 2nd stanza, line 3). The poet constructs a soulful natural environment, which became part of the national Romantic construction of "Swedishness". It formed part of nationalist narratives and heritage expressions, around which a Swedish national identity has since then been constructed. Fröding, together with other writers and artists, provided a generic vernacular that the Swedish population (albeit not all, seeing that about 20 percent of Sweden's population has immigrated to Sweden) now recognize and identifies as a nostalgic yearning for a pastoral idyll. Drawing on natural features during name-giving processes is not unique for Ulleråker. Moon, Kearns, and Joseph identify that it is common that former psychiatric hospital areas are named after the natural environment when they are subject to urban development. They claim that this works to produce a distance from madness and from the area's past as a care facility (Moon, Kearns, and Joseph 2015, 73, 84–87, 122–126, 162).

During the urban development process at Ulleråker, a distance from madness was further provided by drawing on the positive aspects of mental distress. An example of this can be seen in the name-giving process, where Uppsala Municipality's states that "Creativity, madness and genius have a close relationship" (Uppsala kommun 2019, my translation), and in terms of that Fröding's creativity was commemorated through the street names. Drawing on aspects of creativity is not unproblematic as it builds on sanist discourses. James Kaufman and Maureen Neihart explains that the connection between creativity and madness builds on old stereotypes dating back to at least the 1700s when the association between male poets and madness emerged in the Western imaginary. Since that time, a connection between male poets and sensitivity, eccentric behaviour, genius, and madness have been made not only in cultural productions but also in research and in medical and psychological practices (Kaufman 2005, 99; Neihart 1998, 47). Consequently, madness was connected to creative people as well as researchers, psychiatrists, and psychologists. The general public even expected creative people to exhibit madness (Neihart 1998, 47). The idea has lived on, and today researchers claim that they can prove that people diagnosed with, for instance, schizophrenia (as well as their siblings) are overrepresented in creative occupations, and that there is a genetic explanation for their creativity/madness (Kyaga et al. 2011). Since creativity is held as something positive, this discourse works to create some patients, like Fröding, as active citizens contributing to social life. This also makes them far removed from the negative stereotypes of madness that cast patients as irrational, emotive, and dependent.

I suggest that the focus on creativity, as articulated by Uppsala Municipality, does not primarily commemorate Fröding's life and his experiences of being hospitalized. On the contrary, I suggest that it memorializes the Swedish literary world in which Fröding has played and continues to play a prominent role. Fröding is part of the Swedish literary canon and commonly described as one of Sweden's foremost poets; he is credited with continuing, but also modernizing, the Swedish Romantic tradition. Although this may seem positive, Rita Felski reminds us that it is important to remain critical of literary canons as they, with very few exceptions, are limited to the work of white heterosexual men from privileged positions in society (Felski 2003, 12–22, 64–71). Fröding is no exception; he was from the intellectual upper-middle class and moved in circles of powerful men who supported his authorship (Brandell 2019). It has been noted that literature incorporated into canons is often chosen and furthered by groups of white powerful men (Felski 2003, 12–22, 64–71). Building on this, I suggest that the street names do not primarily memorialise the patient Fröding but the Swedish literary canon and, by extension, the street names work to commemorate a hegemonic discourse about male homosociality. More importantly, they memorialise ideas of male genius in line with prevailing ideas about gendered giftedness. As such, the street names can be considered an extension and reproduction of gendered upper-middle-class ideologies that remain pervasive and persistent not only in name-giving processes but also in cultural heritage at large.

5   Street Names that Leak Experiences of Madness

Nevertheless, if we consider street names as a medium through which narratives are realized (Ryan, Foote, and Azaryahu 2016, 158–159), it is also possible that the street names mediate other stories. Exploring this, I examine how the street names – Bergtrollsvägen (Mountain Troll Street), Fylgiavägen (Fylgia

Street), Levnadsfärden (The Journey of Life), Morgondrömsvägen (Morning Dream Street) – *leak* Fröding's very personal experience of madness, particularly his experiences of exclusion, alcoholism, depression, and addiction to sexual services. The street names also *leak* Fröding's critique of medical practices and social norms during the turn of the twentieth century.

To explain this, I start by discussing the street name Bergtrollsvägen (Mountain troll street), which alludes to one of Fröding's best-known poems, "Ett gammalt bergtoll" ("An Old Mountain Troll"), from the collection *Splashes and Patches* (1999 [1896]). In the poem, the reader sees the world through the eyes of a troll. It begins with the troll stating that he should really return to the mountain where he lives "but in the dale here it is just right" and "it is so good were people dwell" (Fröding 1999, 34. 1st stanza, line 4, and 2nd stanza, line 3). The troll wants to linger in the dale but at the same time experiences that he does not belong there. This is a common depiction of trolls in Nordic literature where, according to Ann-Sofie Lönngren (2015, 218), they are characterized as strangers in the human world and as bodies out of place. This is also depicted in what Fröding further writes,

> The rabble keeps out of reach now
> and point their fingers, safe from afar,
> and run off and loudly screech now:
> Ugh! what a bad troll you are!
>> FRÖDING 1999 [1896], 34, 4th stanza, lines 1–4

The poem depicts children shouting abusive words and pointing fingers from afar, not wanting to be too close to the troll. The verse makes visible, in a very painful manner, strategies of othering and of exclusion. It shows a form of stereotypical mapping of the self and the other, where the distance – not wanting to be close to the troll – functions as means to maintain boundaries between the self (humans) and the other (trolls). The production and maintenance of these symbolic boundaries work to deny the troll a belonging in the dale that he so much desires.

Ethnologist Ebbe Schön argues that the poem is a depiction of Fröding's own life and of his experiences of feeling and being socially deviant (1991, 31). For Fröding and others diagnosed with "mental illness", or those who in one way or the other did not live up to social norms, the matter of belonging was (and is) a very real issue. The medical community was instrumental in maintaining boundaries of belonging by pointing out those who transgressed these boundaries and implementing efforts to adjust behaviours as well as uphold social norms. The boundaries established by this community took material

shape in the form of psychiatric hospitals, physically removing people diagnosed with "mental illness" from other social spaces and placing them in these
secluded places. Thus, it is possible to read the mountain as a metaphor for the
psychiatric hospital, and the dale as the society outside the hospital.

The troll's otherness is also expressed in the description of his ugliness, seen
especially when he encounters a sweet princess:

> But she was sweet-eyed and mild-eyed
> and looked kind at me, clumsy old cuss,
> though I look evil and wild-eyed
> and her friends fled away from us.
>
> FRÖDING 1999 [1896], 34 5th stanza, lines 1–4

The description of the troll draws on a common negative characterization
of trolls seen in Nordic folklore. In this tradition, trolls embody strength,
stupidity, and clumsiness, which function to dichotomize wilderness (trolls)
and civilization (humans). Trolls are further depicted as something comical
but also as repulsive (Lönngren 2015, 209–211). I suggest that the characterization of the troll as off-putting and ugly makes reference to how mental distress
was described and depicted in 1800's society. At the time, ugliness was considered "a symbolic reflection of the inner state of patients", and the uglier a person was, the more severe the mental distress (Gilman 1995, 36). Thus, the troll
could be read as a symbolic reflection of how society viewed people diagnosed
with "mental illness".

The connection between mental distress and ugliness also materializes in
Fylgiavägen (Fylgia Street) named after the poem "Fylgia" ("Fylgia") from the
collection *New Poems* (Fröding 1998 [1894]). A fylgia is a protective spirit in the
Nordic mythology who appears in dreams and can give premonitions of a person's impending death. However, the poem is not a tale about dying but one of
unhappy love. Fröding writes,

> Fylgia, O, Fylgia, from me do not flee
> when I'm drowned in despair by hot passion's sea,
> you timid one, noble one, shun not my plight
> when with base thoughts I gaze on your pure chaste sight,
> which hovers in beauty and starlight clear
> and you in my deepest dreams appear.
> So near me you are
> but yet too, too far,
>
> FRÖDING 1998 [1894], 83, 1st stanza, lines 1–8

Fylgia refers to Olivia Petersson (m. Rickman) who worked in a restaurant at
the Masonic Lodge in the Swedish town of Karlstad (Furuland 2008). Fröding
was a frequent guest at this restaurant, where he fell in love with Olivia and
proposed. Her parents deemed him unfit to be a husband because he suffered from alcoholism, and because of this she rejected his proposal (Furuland
2008; Cullberg 2004, 65–69). Consuming large amounts of alcohol was common at the time in Sweden, but Fröding's substantial alcohol intake resulted
in delirium and diabetes, and he was hospitalized at psychiatric care facilities
several times for the negative effects alcoholism had on him (Cullberg 2004,
35–49, 54). However, it was not the physical effects of alcoholism that deemed
Fröding unfit for marriage but the connection between alcoholism and mental
distress that was made in the 1800's society and in medical practices. Being
an alcoholic was considered a sign of a lack of morals, a trait of a degenerated
human being, and, consequently, pathologized (Johannisson 1990, 130, 150).
Moreover, alcoholism was largely associated with the poorest in society, and,
at the time, being poor was in many cases equated with being less mentally
capable (Johannisson 1990, 150).

I suggest that the street name Fylgiavägen *leaks* experiences of madness,
maybe more so in the Swedish original version of the poem, where the phrase
"when I'm drowned in despair by hot passion's sea" ("när jag drags av det låga
mot dyn") can be translated more literally to "when I am dragged by the base-
ness down into the mire". Although base needs can refer to passion, it could
also mean being dragged down by alcohol or by depression. In the poem
"base thoughts" (lumpna tankar), sexual thoughts or thoughts brought on by
depression and/or alcohol, threaten Fylgia's "pure chaste sight, which hov-
ers in beauty and starlight clear". The underpinning message in this poem is
the juxtaposition of beauty/health and baseness/illness, where the presence
or proximity to the protagonist threatens to project baseness/"illness" onto
Fylgia's pure image.

"Fylgia" and "An Old Mountain Troll" are poems about love and focus on
the contrast between the innocent, that which Fröding's protagonists do
not possess but constantly seek, and the ugly, that which Fröding's protagonists embody. These themes run through Fröding's poetry, together with
the theme of sexuality. The latter theme is materialized through the street
Morgondrömsvägen, named after the poem "En morgondröm" ("A Morning
Dream") from the collection *Splashes and Patches* (Fröding 1999 [1896]).
"A Morning Dream" alludes to a dreamlike state that appears just before wak-
ing up, which Germund Michanek calls a "dream of happiness", a dream about
the happiest time in life (Michanek 1962, 152–158). I would argue that this is a
quite chaste interpretation and that it should rather be understood as an erotic

and orgasmic dream, seeing that Fröding describes heterosexual intercourse, which ends with the man orgasming inside the woman. Fröding writes,

> And like Arien's rosebud one spring of old
> her veiling pink petals from pistils unfold
> before sun, winds and seeds in the air
> she lay naked and in bloom so fair
> and with soft trembling breasts, knees wide spread she invited
> that their loving desire be united.

> Soul aflame and blood now stirs,
> she was his and he was hers,
> he was she, she was he,
> one and both elated,
> when his firm manhood you see
> in her penetrated.

> And with head leaning backward in kissing's fierce lust
> and with bosom 'gainst embracing thrust,
> she drank living and love's finest drink, all the same
> in each spurting that came
> of his hot life's juice,
> in each sparking and flame
> his powers produce.
>
> FRÖDING 1999 [1896], 53, 18th–20th stanza, lines 1–6

Poets of his time avoided frank depictions of heterosexual intercourse, and this poem would come to create problems for Fröding. He was charged with sexual offence in court, and although he was eventually freed, the poem was only printed in its entirety in 1955, almost 60 years after it was first released (Michanek 1962, 23, 190, 259–297).

The street Morgondrömsvägen should not only be understood as narrating erotic experiences but also as *leaking* experiences of madness. It can be read as a critique of how a Swedish Christian society viewed and delimited sexuality and a critique of psychiatric practices during the turn of the twentieth century. Karin Johannisson (1990, 126–156) explains that during the late 1800's, norms concerning sexuality were characterized by moderation and self-control. Sexual activities were not only supposed to be controlled but also delimited (Johannisson 1990, 150). The poem's uninhibited exploration of heterosexual intercourse certainly goes against this norm. Moreover, the poem makes several references to Fröding's own life and his sexual desires. To begin with, Fröding was addicted to sexual services provided by prostitutes (Michanek 1962, 49–55; Cullberg 2004, 35–49, 54). Visiting prostitutes was normalized at the time, and reveals more about the patriarchal society Fröding lived in than of his sexuality. However, his addiction to sexual services and his seeming inability to control and moderate his sexual desires were behaviours labelled as "mental illness" at the time (see Johannisson 1990, 150). Fröding also openly, in the text "bikt" ("Confession"), which was sent to the school teacher Edvard Walentin Gelin together with a letter asking him to read the confession out loud in church, articulates an interest in masturbation, fornication (sodomy) and sadomasochism (Michanek 1992, 110; Cullberg 2004, 92–94). These desires were considered sexual promiscuity, and according to Johannisson, seen as akin to alcoholism. As mentioned above, alcoholism was at the time associated with the poorest in society and connected to a lack of morals. Moreover, fornication was punishable by law (Johannisson 1990, 150).

The street Levnadsfärden ("The Journey of Life"), which takes its name from the poem of the same name from the book *Splashes from the Grail* (Fröding 1998 [1894]), can be understood in a similar manner. In "The Journey of Life" Fröding depicts a life journey of a heterosexual couple,

> Gentle destinies,
> Suffer through
> harsh destinies
> taking, giving,
> to be enlivened, alive
>
> FRÖDING 1998 [1894], 82, first stanza, lines 9–13, my translation

The poem is a meditation on a monogamous heteronormative temporality and portrays the harshness and gentleness of this kind of life. Towards the end of the poem Fröding asks, "is it not so, oh you wise one, is it not so, the one to us given, the only [life] worth living, the journey of life?" (Fröding 1998 [1894], 82, 2nd stanza, lines 20–23, my translation). These lines hold a certain ambiguity, because, on the one hand, it is a story about Adam and Eve, the fall of man and the loss of Eden, which relates to the set of Christian morals concerning sexuality. As such it establishes that a Christian moral conduct and a heteronormative life is the only life worth living. On the other hand, the lines open up to a reading where the heteronormative life path is questioned: is it the only life worth living?

Questioning the validity of a heteronormative life can be read as a critique of late-1800's medical discourses concerning sexuality and madness. Sexuality was a central aspect in diagnosing "mental illness" during the 1880's. Johannisson writes that there was a Christian ideal that the body was not supposed to become a slave to its desires and that human existence must be characterized by morality, reason, and control. This applied to relations not only outside of wedlock but also within marriage (Johannisson 1990, 130). At the time, medical practitioners categorized non-reproductive sexuality, including homosexuality and sadomasochism, as "psychopatia", a pathological category used to diagnose so-called abnormal behaviour as well as a term used to describe a degenerated human type (Johannisson 1990, 130; Johannisson 2015, 25–27). Moreover, deviant sexual behaviour was considered to produce unhealthy offspring, and, consequently, sterilization and marriage prohibition were thought to be appropriated in order to control and secure a healthy population (Johannisson 1990, 140–143). The narratives in the poem "A Morning Dream" (as well as Fröding's own lifestyle) transgressed many of the boundaries of what was considered normative, and the narrative in the poem "The Journey of Life" calls monogamous heteronormativity into question. Considering that the streets Morgondrömsvägen and Levnadsfärden hold these narratives allows for them to mediate a critique of social norms, both of heterosexuality and of the late 1800's psychiatry and medical sciences that stigmatized non-reproductive sexual expressions in the urban landscape.

6   Conclusion

In this article, I have conducted two different kinds of mad readings. First, I focus on the name-giving process of streets and explore how sanist discourses permeates this process. I discuss what histories are furthered and what heritage this produces. Second, I focus on mad leakages. Connecting the street names to the poems that gave them their names, and further connecting them to Fröding's life and experience of madness as well as to medical discourses and social norms at the time, I expose stories about madness that the street names hold. Thus, I participate in creating a mad heritage for Ulleråker.

The first part of this article shows that street naming is closely connected to Uppsala Municipality's conceptualization of the place as articulated during the urban development, and to local and national heritage politics explaining what Uppsala's cultural heritage constitutes. These centre on creativity and favour male historical figures, resulting in street names that predominantly commemorate the Swedish literary canon. I further argue that this process is a celebration of male homosociality and patriarchal values. I suggest that focusing on a former patient's poetry furthers old stereotypes and sanist discourses about the connection between creativity and madness. Within the discourse of cultural heritage, these ideas are now materialized as Ulleråkers cultural heritage. In addition, choosing names for the streets that bring to mind fanciful imaginative mythological landscapes plays on Swedish nationalist narratives. I suggest that a strategic forgetting of madness is realized at Ulleråker. The street naming at Ulleråker works as a form of rebranding of the former psychiatric hospital area, where certain versions of the pasts are used to create more happy futures.

At the same time, the municipal officials were instrumental in assuring a remembrance of a previous patient's accomplishments when suggesting the street names. This can be seen as a negotiation of dominant discourses in an attempt to commemorate pain, addiction, anxiety, depression, and non-heteronormative sexual desires as well as to include madness in the post-asylum landscape. Yet, for madness to *leak* into urban landscapes, efforts need to be made to find and open up the *cracks* so as to allow these stories to seep out and be visible in the streets. Chances are that the street names will only be seen as fanciful names if the stories of madness are not told. Here mad reading can play a role in the future narrative of the post-asylum landscape since the method is not only a tool to examine how madness emerges but also a way to tell stories of madness.

In this text I show how a mad reading of street names can provide mad narratives for the post-asylum landscape. A mad reading is not only a reading of street names; it is a "doing" of cultural heritage on par with other heritage practices. This means that the researchers have the possibility to make new connections and suggest other possible stories for the place and the past, which, in turn, can offer promises for other possible futures for the post-asylum landscape. This perspective on mad readings holds the researcher accountable for the stories they tell about the place and makes them active participants in the cultural heritage production. Consequently, a mad reading asks the researcher not only to trouble sanist norms and discourses but also to show how histories can be told differently. Thus, a mad reading is not only an analytic tool but a call for researchers to work towards a more multifaceted cultural heritage.

Acknowledgments

This study forms part of the project *From Psychiatric Hospital to Condominium – Urban Development and Cultural Heritage* (2020–2023), project no: 2019-00589, funded by FORMAS – the research council for sustainable development.

Thanks to the editors, the anonymous peer-reviewer, and Jenny Björklund for valuable comments.

References

Azaryahu, Maoz. 1996. "The Power of Commemorative Street Names." *Environment and Planning D: Society and Space* 14, no. 3 (June): 311–30.

Azaryahu, Maoz. 2012. "Renaming the Past in Post-Nazi Germany: Insights into the Politics of Street Naming in Mannheim and Potsdam." *Cultural Geographies* 19, no. 3 (July): 385–400.

Beckman-Thoor, Karin, and Liselott Blombäck. 2014. Uppsala stad C 40 A. *Riksintresseområde för kulturmiljövården. Fördjupat kunskapsunderlag.* Länsstyrelsens Meddelandeserie. Länsstyrelsen i Uppsala län: Uppsala. www.lansstyrelsen.se/downlo ad/18.4e0415ee166afb593248985/1541146613657/2014-01%20Uppsala%20stad%20 C40A%20Riksintresse%20f%C3%B6r%20kulturmilj%C3%B6v%C3%A5rden%20 -%20f%C3%B6rdjupat%20kunskapsunderlag.pdf.

Brandell, Gunnar. 2019. "Gustaf Fröding." *Svenskt biografiskt lexikon.* Riksarkivet. https://sok.riksarkivet.se/sbl/artikel/14556.

Cullberg, Johan. 2004. *Gustaf Fröding och kärleken: en psykologisk och psykiatrisk studie.* Stockholm: Natur och kultur.

Duminy, James. 2017. "Street Renaming, Symbolic Capital, and Resistance in Durban, South Africa." In *The Political Life of Urban Streetscapes: Naming, Politics, and Place,* edited by Reuben Rose-Redwood, Derek Alderman, and Maoz Azaryahu, 240–258. London and New York: Routledge.

Felski, Rita. 2003. *Literature after Feminism.* Chicago: University of Chicago Press.

Fröding, Gustaf. 1997 [1891]. "Titania," *Guitar and Concertina. Poems by Gustaf Fröding. A new Translation by Mike McArthur.* Winthringham, Malton: The Oak Tree Press, 61.

Fröding, Gustaf. 1998 [1894]. "The Journey of Life," *New Poems. Poems by Gustaf Fröding. A new Translation by Mike McArthur.* Winthringham, Malton: The Oak Tree Press, 82.

Fröding, Gustaf. 1998 [1894] "Fylgia," *New Poems. Poems by Gustaf Fröding. A new Translation by Mike McArthur.* Winthringham, Malton: The Oak Tree Press, 83.

Fröding, Gustaf. 1999 [1896]. "An Old Mountain Troll," *Splashes and Patches. Poems by Gustaf Fröding. A new Translation by Mike McArthur.* Winthringham, Malton: The Oak Tree Press, 34–35.

Fröding, Gustaf. 1999 [1896]. "A Morning Dream," *Splashes and Patches. Poems by Gustaf Fröding. A new Translation by Mike McArthur.* Winthringham, Malton: The Oak Tree Press, 53.

Furuland, Gunel. 2008. "Louise Ekelund & Lars O. Lundgren, Gustaf Fröding och Vackra Vivi. svt: s villfarelser–och verkligheten: Proprius förlag." *Samlaren: tidskrift för svensk litteraturvetenskaplig forskning* 129: 442–443.

Gill, Graeme. 2005. Changing Symbols: The Renovation of Moscow Place Names. *The Russian Review* 64, no. 3 (July): 480–503.

Gilman, Sander. L. 1995. *Health and Illness: Images of Difference*. London: Reaktion Books.

Högström, Ebba. 2018. "'It Used to be Here But Moved Somewhere Else': Post-Asylum Spatialisations – a New Urban Frontier?" *Social and Cultural Geography* 19, no 3 (August): 314–335.

Jonsson, Eva. 2002. *Hospitaltidens lyrik: textkritisk edition av Gustaf Frödings lyriska produktion dec. 1898 - mars 1905*. Uppsala: Uppsala Universitet.

Johannisson, Karin. 1990. *Medicinens öga: sjukdom, medicin och samhälle - historiska erfarenheter*. Stockholm: Norstedt.

Johannisson, Karin. 2015. *Den sårade divan: om psykets estetik (och om Agnes von K, Sigrid H och Nelly S)*. Stockholm: Bonnier.

Kaufman, James C. 2005. "The Door That Leads Into Madness: Eastern European Poets and Mental Illness." *Creativity Research Journal* 17, no. 1 (June): 99–103.

Kearns, Robin Alun Joseph, and Graham Moon. 2012. "Traces of the New Zealand Psychiatric Hospital: Unpacking the Place of Stigma." *New Zealand Geographer* 68, no. 3 (December): 175–186.

Kyaga, Simon, Paul Lichtenstein, Marcus Boman, Christina Hultman, Niklas Långström and Michael Landén. 2011. "Creativity and Mental Disorder: Family Study of 300 000 People with Severe Mental Disorder". *The British Journal of Psychiatry* 199, no. 5 (January): 373–379.

Lantmäteriet. 2016. *Good Place-Name Practice. The Swedish Place-Names Advisory Board's Guide to the Standardisation and Preservation of Place-Names*. Accessable: https://www.lantmateriet.se/contentassets/41a7acabed464c519755771a3b760b84/ortnamn_och_namnvard_nr6_engelsk.pdf

LeFrançois, Brenda, Robert Menzies, and Geoffrey Reaume. 2013. "Glossary of Terms". In *Mad Matters: a Critical Reader in Canadian Mad Studies*, edited by Brenda LeFrançois, Robert Menzies and Geoffrey Reaume, 334–341. Toronto: Canadian Scholar's Press Inc.

Light, Duncan. 2004. "Street names in Bucharest, 1990–1997: Exploring the Modern Historical Geographies of Post-Socialist Change".*Journal of Historical Geography* 30, no. 1 (January): 154–172.

Light, Duncan, and Craig Young. 2014. "Habit, Memory, and the Persistence of Socialist-Era Street Names in Postsocialist Bucharest, Romania". *Annals of the Association of American Geographers* 104, no. 3, (April): 668–685.

Lönngren, Ann-Sofie. 2015. "Trolls!! Folklore, literature and 'othering.'" In *Rethinking National Literatures and the Literary Canon in Scandinavia*, edited by Ann-Sofie Lönngren, Heidi Grönstrand, Dag Heede and Anne Heith, 205–230. Newcastle: Cambridge Scholars Publishing.

McRuer, Robert. 2019. "In Focus: Cripping Cinema and Media Studies: Introduction." *Journal of Cinema and Media Studies* 58, no. 4 (Summer): 134–139.

Michanek, Germund. 1962. *En morgondröm: studier kring Frödings ariska dikt.* Uppsala: Uppsala universitet.

Michanek, Germund. 1992. *Från Frödings värld.* Höganäs: Wiken.

Moon, Graham, Robin Kearns, and Alun Joseph. 2015. *The Afterlives of the Psychiatric Asylum: Recycling Concepts, Sites and Memories.* Farnham, Surrey: Ashgate.

Municipal official. 2018. Personal communication with Cecilia Rodéhn via e-mail 2018–06–28.

Namngivningsnämnden. 2016a. Sammanställningen av medborgarförslag på namn i Ulleråker inkomna våren 2016. Accessed via a municipal official.

Namngivningsnämndens arbetsutskott. 2016. Namngivningsnämndens arbetsutskott. 2016–09–05 § 40 Namn på vägar i centrala Ulleråker NGN-2016-0021, §45 Namn på kvarter, vägar och torg i Centrala Ulleråker NGN-2016-0021. §46 Namn på kvarter och park i Ulleråker, parker vid vattentornet NGN-2016-0022. Dnr: NGN-2016-0022.

Neihart, Maureen. 1998. "Creativity, the Arts, and Madness." *Roeper Review* 21, no.1 (January): 47–50.

Palonen, Emilia. 2008. "The City-Text in Post-Communist Budapest: Street Names, Memorials, and the Politics of Commemoration." *GeoJournal* 73, no. 3 (September): 219–230.

Rodéhn, Cecilia. 2022. "Introducing Mad Studies and Mad Reading to Game Studies." *Game Studies* 22 (1):1–15.

Ryan, Marie-Laure, Kenneth E. Foote, and Maoz Azaryahu. 2016. *Narrating Space, Spatializing Narrative: Where Narrative Theory and Geography Meet.* Columbus: The Ohio State University Press.

Sandow, Elin. 2016. "Hennes jobb: Ge namn till gator och torg." *Upsala Nya Tidning* 2016, 10, 07, 10.

Schön, Ebbe. 1991. Folkets sångmö: Nittiotalisterna och folkkulturen. I 90-*tal Visioner och Vägval Nordiska museet och Skansens årsbok. Fataburen*, edited by Hans Medelius and Sten Rentzhog, 19–43. Stockholm: Nordiska Museet.

Shoval, Noam. 2013. "Street-naming, tourism development and cultural conflict: the case of the Old City of Acre/Akko/Akka." *Transactions of the Institute of British Geographers* 38, no. 4 (October): 612–626.

Smith, Laurajane. 2006. *Uses of Heritage.* New York and London: Routledge.

Stadsbyggnadsförvaltningen. 2016. Förslag: Namn på kvarter och park i Ulleråker, parker vid vattentornet, daterad 2016–06–28. Dnr: NGN-2016-0022. Accessed via a municipal offical 2016–06–29.

Uppsala kommun 2019. Historiskt ankare i det nya Ulleråker. 2019–02–15. https://bygg .uppsala.se/for-byggaktorer/hospitalet/bakgrund-till-tavlingen/historiskt-ankare-i -det-nya-ulleraker/ (accessed July 07, 2019).

Wanjiru, Melissa Wangui, and Kosuke Matsubara. 2017. "Street Toponymy and the Decolonisation of the Urban Landscape in Post-Colonial Nairobi." *Journal of Cultural Geography* 34, no.1 (July): 1–23.

Winberg, Charlotte. 2018. Här är förslagen på de nya gatunamnen. *Upsala Nya tidning* 2018, 08, 01, 10.

Wolframe, PhebeAnn M. 2014. *Reading Through Madness: Counter-Psychiatric Epistemologies and the Biopolitics of (In) sanity in Post-World War II Anglo Atlantic Women's Narratives* (Doctoral dissertation). Hamilton: McMaster University.

CHAPTER 8

Normality Narrative in the Context of the Lunatic Rights Movement

Tomke Hinrichs

Abstract

Around 1900, German psychiatry was in a transition phase. To gain the necessary acceptance from science and also from society, the young medical discipline had to establish itself. Psychiatric patients were supposed to comply with the diagnosis they received from their doctors. But some of them didn't and tried to obtain society's support in their own way. I examine the situation of psychiatry and the handling of people, who became "psychiatrised" – meaning people who unwillingly became subject to psychiatric treatments. The focus lies on cases, which are relevant in the context of the lunatic rights movement from the 1890s onwards, where the affected persons were trying to obtain their rights and citizenship back, because they did not only lose certain civil rights, but also were mostly 'processed' as objects during the treatment.

Writing pamphlets was one option for patients to try and convince a broader public that they were, in fact, not lunatic. In these pamphlets, they told about their diagnosis and the experiences they had made in asylum. Furthermore, they submitted petitions to some parliaments to get their civil rights back. My research focuses on how these persons were reificated as objects and how they tried to return to themselves/their selves as subjects.

A more extensive question is here the question of normality. Since this enables the writers to find their way into society, they use it as an argument. The normality narrative is the core of my thesis. Some questions are: What does normal mean? How do they try to explain that they are normal? To be "normal" was their way back into society. It meant that they are healthy – not mentally ill – they could be a "normal" member of the society.

In this article I would like to reconstruct some cases and to point out how the writers try to show within the brochures how normal they are. Some questions will be: Which argumentation did they use? Are there similarities to each other? Are there some connections between the different cases?

Keywords

abuse – biography – bourgeois death – German psychiatry around 1900 – incapacitation – lunatic rights movement – normality narrative – normal/regular – healthy – pamphlets (dt. Irrenbroschüren) – perception – recognition – self-empowerment – subjectivation – troublemaker insanity (dt. Querulantenwahnsinn) – women's movement

1   Definition Narrative

In this article I use a literary definition of narrative from the narrative theories of Monika Fludernik and Marie-Laure Ryan, which allows me to access the narratives found in the examined lunatics brochures. According to Fludernik and Ryan, a text can be classified as a narrative if it contains reporting sequences or describes sequences or events (Fludernik and Ryan 2020, 7–10). These sequences must take place at a certain point in time in certain places and must represent temporal sequences. The focus is thus on a narrative that is seen as a report of chains of events.[1] Fludernik and Ryan propose three different kinds of narrativity. In case of the narratives examined below one could classify these as strong narratives. A strong narrative does not end with the depiction of sequences and includes "[...] mental worlds of human [...], on their desires, intentions and feelings." (Fludernik and Ryan 2020, 9). The authors of the brochures aim to influence and convince readers of their 'normal' health. Therefore, these authors compile a chain of events in their respective lives. The biographical aspects serve to show how healthy or *normal* they are. The authors use a similar argumentation, through which they are connected to each other, as all of them pursue the same goal of rehabilitation. They prepare a story or a report with the help of their own biography and create the source material for my analysis and the object of investigation of the normality narrative.

---

1 German Research Foundation (DFG) Research Training Group 1767 'Factual and Fictional Narrative' at the University of Freiburg under the direction of Prof. Dr. Monika Fludernik. Research Program of the Research Training Group "Factual and Fictional Narrative. Differences, Interferences and Congruencies in Narratological Perspective", online in: http://www.grk-erzaehlen.uni-freiburg.de/wp-content/uploads/2014/05/grk1767-forschung.pdf, 2, 3; (accessed August 24, 2020), https://www.grk-erzaehlen.uni-freiburg.de/english-summary/ (accessed September 22, 2020).

2   The Normality Narrative in the Context of the Lunatic Rights
       Movement

Around 1900, German psychiatry was in a transition phase. To gain the necessary acceptance from science and also from society, the young medical discipline had to establish itself. Psychiatric patients were supposed to comply with
the diagnosis they received from their doctors. Yet some of them did not and
tried to obtain society's support in their own way. I examine the situation of
psychiatry and the handling of people who became "psychiatrised" – people
who unwillingly became subject to psychiatric treatments. The focus lies on
cases which are relevant in the context of the lunatic rights movement from
the 1890s onwards, in which those affected attempted to regain their rights
and citizenship, as this 'disenfranchisement' could go as far as the loss of civil
rights. During this treatment they were mostly 'processed' as objects. Writing
pamphlets was one option for patients to try and convince a broader public
that they were, in fact, not lunatics. In these pamphlets, they wrote about their
diagnoses and the experiences they had made in asylums. Furthermore, they
submitted petitions to some parliaments to regain their civil rights. My research
focuses on how these persons were reified as objects, or as "ill" subjects and
thus how they tried to convince the public for them to be acknowledged as and
referred to as healthy subjects.

   Through this, a more fundamental question is raised. The question of
normality or rather who defines normality. The writers use normality as an
argument since this enables them to find their way back into society. They
see themselves as healthy and therefore claim their right to be a *normal/regu-
lar* member of society. Cornelia Brink is pursuing a research approach in her
habilitation thesis which is similar to mine. She writes about normalities as
patterns of interpretation and narrative strategies in the context of a social and
cultural history of psychiatry. I, on the other hand, will use a micro-historical
depth cut and reconstruct the cases with additional archival sources, such as
medical records etc. with a focus on subjectivity. I use Subjectivation as follows: Subjectivation in this context means full recognition and autonomy
of a person or institution in its relationship to the environment as an acting
subject. Additionally, I will include the aspect of recognition in the problem,
which can also be found in the beginnings of psychiatry (see Brink 2010). The
lack of recognition can be found in the context of the emergence of the new
psychiatric discipline as a new medical discipline in its own right in the middle of the nineteenth century. At the beginning, it was not recognised as an
independent discipline. The normality narrative is at the core of my thesis.
The central questions are: What does normal mean? How do the writers claim,

try to explain and justify to be accepted as normal? In this chapter I will reconstruct two cases and analyse the urge to be recognised as normal through the writing of pamphlets. The analysis will focus on similarities within the strategies of writing and connections between their cases.

3   Thematic Framing

More than 100 years ago, admission to a psychiatric institution in most cases equalled the loss of membership in society. Psychiatry was in a state of upheaval around 1900. The young medical discipline had to establish itself in order to gain the necessary acceptance from science and society. Yet there were protests against psychiatry expressed by various social groups. German psychiatry today can only be understood when viewed in this context. It has been questioned ever since the beginning of psychiatry whether it is to be recognized as a true medical discipline. Hence diagnoses have been questioned, especially by several reform movements. These include the lunatic rights movement from the 1890s into the 1920s and the reform efforts in the 1960s, whose implementation for improvement within psychiatric structures lasted until the 1990s (see Schmiedebach 1996; Fangerau and Nolte 2006).

The period of the Third Reich is excluded here, because of the politically dominated circumstances. The lunatic rights movement around 1900 is special because in this movement, psychiatrised or people with a mental distress first spoke up for themselves and joined forces. They made themselves "experts in their own field. [transl., T. H.]" (Schmuhl 2009, 7–9). Well over 200 patients made their experiences of and about psychiatric diagnoses and interventions public, a first time ever event.[2]

Until then psychiatric patients were supposed to comply with the diagnosis and the interventions they received. Yet some of them did not and tried to obtain society's support in their own way. They tried to revise the diagnoses made by the doctors and to restore, consolidate or renew their standing in society. Their brochures or protest leaflets were the basis of the lunatic rights movement and were primarily directed against claimed abuses and abuse by the psychiatric system itself. The demands of the lunatic rights movement, which were first reflected in the so-called lunatic pamphlets, were primarily

---

2   For the number of 200 pamphlets (see Brink 2002, 24); for collections of the lunatic brochures (see Beyer 1912).

aimed at eliminating the abuses in the procedures for incapacitation, turned against the common practice of incarceration and the prevailing conditions in the institutions (Schmiedebach 1996, 156). Another focus of these protests was the proof of a 'regular' life, in order to be able to shed the *bourgeois death* (Bernet 2007) suffered through diagnosis or admission to an institution. This was of course linked to the issue of fundamental rights and freedoms, which were curtailed in the context of psychiatric treatment. This legal restriction applied in particular to citizenship and civic status, as this was often revoked at the point of admission to a psychiatry. Without these rights, an active participation and involvement in social life was impossible. Not only did the social conditions change for the individual concerned, but also his or her personal environment beyond the family could be afflicted. In summary, there was a lack of acceptance for the discipline of psychiatry. My presumption is that firstly, psychiatry was not fully subjectivated as a medical discipline. Secondly, the instrument of psychiatry and several other disciplines – the diagnoses – had to fight for acceptance. Thirdly, the doctors were not accepted. And at last, on the *fourth* level, the patient, who is addressed as "lunatic", refused this and tried to subjectivate herself or himself with the help of a pamphlet. In this the writers of the brochures demonstrate: "I am as normal as the others!" They tried to reach society, which was supposed to judge by means of common sense, if these patients were healthy or ill.

The German word *Irrenbroschüre* can be translated as a lunatic brochure. On a psychiatric conference in Göttingen on 21st November 1894, a speaker called these pamphlets 'brochures' (*Broschüren*) and afterwards the writers where called *Broschürenschreiber*, meaning 'writers of brochures'. As a result, the brochures were called *Irrenbroschüren* because its writers were being labelled as mentally ill/lunatic ("*Irre*") (Kirchheim 1895). This leads to the problem that these brochures are not listed in a library catalogue as books published by persons labelled as mentally ill. To detect these sources, I have identified three conditions: *Firstly*, the authors of the pamphlets deny to be "mentally ill"; *Secondly*, they criticise the situation in the asylum (for example: abuse, overcrowding); *Thirdly*, they table reform proposals to improve the situation regarding imprisonment or procedure of incapacitation.

This chapter focuses on the narratives of the authors of the pamphlets and the *normality narratives* to which they refer in the pamphlets. Therefore, this chapter presents aspects that belong to the *normality narrative* from the brochures. I will focus on the self and the constitution of the self in a reconstruction of these cases in my doctoral thesis. This part is left out here.

4   Normal and the Normality Narrative

To understand what *normal/regular*[3] means, it is important to define this term. It is therefore mandatory to take a closer look at the source of the word, which lies in the Greek language, and acknowledge that *normal* is closely interwoven with some other concepts. The *first* term is "nature" (Kudlien and Ritter 1984, 920) which is a reference value for regular things and the natural constitution (Gemoll 1991, 795). 'Nature' means – particularly in the Hippocratic writings – on the one hand, the average 'natural' condition, on the other hand, for instance, the healthy condition of the body and its organs and thus the ideal condition whose restoration is the aim of medical treatment [transl., T. H.]" (Kudlien and Ritter 1984, 920). Secondly, the term *normal* is closely interwoven with "healthy". The normal condition is a special medical norm (*ibid.*) This clearly emphasizes the connection between normal, nature, and healthy. This brings us closer to someone who behaves "right", i.e. according to the norms. The translations from the Greek underline the link with the behaviour: It means "just". Besides, these translations are also to be assigned to it, for example "well-ordered", "regular", "civilised" or "well-balanced", to name but a few.[4] They indicate the reference to balanced and "good" behaviour and nature as a scale (Hofmann and Schrader 1984, 906). Thus the guiding idea of "[...] nature, which is the norm of the law [...]. [transl., T. H.]" is obvious (*ibid.*). Nature – health – behaviour are set in a relative frame. This shows that the word points to something "conforming to rules [transl., T. H.]" like civilized behaviour, balance, or a submission or even subordination to certain rules. However, it is important to understand that the meaning of the term *nature* also constantly changes, since it refers to an ideal state which can differ (Kudlien and Ritter 1984, 920).

Subjective perception of their lives plays a major role in this context (Canguilhem 1974, 122). For the individual, the state of health is linked to the normal state, i.e. as soon as the normal can no longer be exercised, there is too much deviation from one's own norm. The boundaries between the two are fluid.

The next step is to define narrative. The definition of narrativity I work with is as stated by Monika Fludernik and Marie-Laure Ryan. They state that a text can be classified as a narrative if it contains reporting sequences or describes sequences or events (Fludernik and Ryan 2020, 7–10). These sequences must

---

3   In the following the term *normal* is used, which could also be translated as *regular*. For reasons of comprehensibility, the technical term is used in the variant that comes closest to German.

4   „δίκαιος" (díkaios) (see Crane 2020).

take place at a certain point in time in certain places and must represent temporal sequences. The focus is thus on a narrative that is seen as a report of chains of events. A further definition, provided again by the authors mentioned above, describes three kinds of narrativity: One strong and two weak kinds of narrative, starting from a basic definition.[5] In the instance of the lunatic brochures it is a strong narrativity. It does not end with the depiction of sequences and includes "[...] mental worlds of human or human-like protagonists [...], on their desires, intentions and feelings." (*ibid*, 9). Moreover "[a]udiences are invited [...] to participate imaginatively and emotionally in the represented events and to immerse themselves in the storyworld." (*ibid*, 9). This narrativity can often be found in "conversational narratives" and in "autobiography" (*ibid*, 9).

When the cases are classified, according to the definitions by Fludernik and Ryan, they are listed as a strong narrativity, because of its compliance with the criteria of the basic definition and the autobiographical features within the brochures of the affected persons (*ibid*, 9–10). One additional aspect is that the authors of the brochures aim to influence and convince the reader of their normal health and therefore compile a chain of events in their own lives. The biographical aspects serve to show how healthy or *normal* they are. In our case it is a strong narrativity, since the affected persons use a similar argumentation through which they are connected to each other, as they pursue the same goal of rehabilitation. They prepare a story or a report with the help of their own biography.

The biography plays, as already mentioned, a major role for the affected persons in their urge to regain widely accepted *normality*. This is evident in their published brochures as well as in the context of keeping a medical record and making a diagnosis. These three aspects have to be investigated carefully. Firstly, applying the concept of the biographical generator formulated by Alois Hahn, one can say that the diagnoses act as biographical generators (Hahn 1987, 12). Without a diagnosis as a trigger, the affected persons would not have felt the need to address in a brochure their "equality" with others in society or the injustice they suffered. The diagnoses discriminate and exclude them. Hahn names institutions that "[...] allow such a return to one's own existence. [transl., T. H.]" as biography generators. As examples he states religious confession, psychoanalysis, the diary, memoirs, medical anamnesis, or confessions in court. Hahn makes a strict distinction between curriculum vitae and biography. For him, curriculum vitae is "[...] a totality of events, experiences,

---

5   (see e.g. Fludernik, and Ryan 2020).

sensations, etc. [...]. [transl., T. H.]". In contrary, the term biography offers infinite possibilities of combination of life events. The individual itself makes the course of life the subject in his biography. By selection alone, a new order of events emerges (Hahn 1987, 12–13). Biography is part of the self-esteem process of individuals (Etzemüller 2012, 48). Secondly, the biography occupies a large space in the medical records – both when creating and continuing the medical record. This was obvious when reviewing the psychiatric medical records. The biographical parts were used for diagnostics. In 1987, Rainer Tölle wrote about the tradition of 'integrating' the biography into the psychiatric medical history to possibly explain the clinical picture (Tölle 1987). Thirdly, biographical aspects were used to try to understand symptoms or give therapeutical approaches matching the biography or breaks in it (Wolter, Beyer, and Lohff 2013). Ulrike Hoffmann-Richter observes: "In a psychiatric patient file, the aim is to obtain the patient's medical history from the biography; to describe and record past and present symptoms as important tools for making a diagnosis. [transl., T. H.]" (Hoffmann-Richter 1995, 205).

The following section describes the method of the analysis. The focus remains on the normality narrative of the authors. Excerpts from the medical records are used to supplement the information in a few points.

5   How to Analyse the Cases?

The cases give a brief insight into the pamphlets and the used *narratives*. Following the thesis of Ann Goldberg, writing a pamphlet was a phenomenon of the bourgeoisie (Tölle 1987). After reviewing various brochures, however, it become evident that it was not just the social class of the bourgeoisie, but any social class that wrote brochures. This is the reason why two cases were chosen for this chapter – that of a wealthy woman coming from an upper-class background and a poorer man of a lower social class.

As shown in the last section, the biography appears as the pivotal point at which the elements of the *normality narrative* become visible in an analysis. I analyse aspects in the narratives that point to an ordinary and regular life. Everyone is socially involved with family, friends and is employed to a certain extend. They lead an orderly life, their days are structured and it seems that everything is well ordered. Therefore, I will use superordinate categories that can be assigned to *normality* such as family, profession, and social life/environment to clarify the *normality narrative*, since all points can be summarized and clarified under these categories. The starting point however is the question of whether the persons concerned doubt their diagnosis.

6   Minor Case Studies

The first case is that of Johann Andreas Rodig. In research, this case is not completely unknown. Two of his brochures are listed everywhere, but during my
research I discovered a third one (Brink 2010, 172). Cornelia Brink mentioned
the case Rodig to point out similarities to other cases in the argumentation,
here about being healthy (*ibid.*, 171–177). Zvi Lothane explains the case of Rodig
while investigating the case of Daniel Paul Schreber[6] and the role of Professor
Flechsig[7] in it (Lothane 1992, 234). Rodig is mentioned as a contemporary of
Schreber and as a case in which Professor Flechsig also played a role.

   The son of the master weaver Johann Christoph Rodig and his wife Sophie
Ottilie was born on July 20, 1850 in Erfurt as one of three children. His case offers
multiple layers, because of several stays in psychiatric institutions and the three
written brochures he has published. I use two patient records, consisting of 19
and 70 pages, and a medical observation report with 12 pages. Furthermore,
I list a number of protocols of the parliament debating his case. Rodig was
officially diagnosed with 'troublemaker insanity' (dt. Querulatenwahnsinn).[8]

   He tries three times to obtain public aid and to rehabilitate himself. This
is indicated by the intervals between the publications in 1896, 1897 and 1902.

---

6   The case of and around Daniel Paul Schreber (1842–1911) is not considered here because of the
    already extensive investigation into his "experience report" and the events that occurred. His
    case became known primarily through Sigmund Freud (1856–1939), who addressed the case
    of Schreber in the context of his studies on psychosis. The "memorabilia of a nervous patient"
    Schrebers exceeds the content of the brochures examined here due to their volume (for more
    information on Schreber see Heiligenthal 1985; Lothane 1992; Santner 1996; Schreber 1973).

7   This refers to Paul Emil Flechsig (1847–1929), a brain researcher and psychiatrist from Leip-
    zig. He was primarily trained in the neurological and pathological fields. Despite a lack of
    training in the psychiatric field, he was selected in 1877/8 to head the building of the new
    psychiatric clinic. He took on a professorship at the psychiatric chair (see, e.g., Steinberg
    2005, 81–120; Lothane 1992).

8   The diagnosis of troublemaker insanity was accompanied by an agreement on accounta-
    bility. The most important result of Ann Goldberg's study is that these cases should not be
    reduced to this diagnosis and that the freedoms of the individual should not be ignored. It
    was precisely with the 'diagnosis' of 'troublemaker insanity' that the research questioned
    the interpretive power of psychiatrists in the case of various authors, who usually acted as
    expert witnesses in court and made their description of the patient's behaviour, which they
    considered deviant, the diagnosis. In contrast, someone with a different diagnosis of men-
    tal distress was denied his rights (Goldberg 2003, 208). For these reasons, the diagnosis had
    been considered an "arbitrary measure and abuse of power by psychiatrists" in the mental
    rights reform movement, and became vulnerable to attack by them because of the unclear
    delineation of this illness (Schwoch and Schmiedebach 2007, 34). Karen Nolte states that
    this diagnosis was "from the beginning closely linked to the social criticism of psychiatric
    institutional therapy" (Nolte 2006, 396).

In his field reports, he describes how he came to the asylum, what happened to him during his stay there and how the short-term development of his life went after his release from the asylum. In doing so, he draws a picture of how the charges and accusations brought against him came about and how he assesses his involvement in them. His descriptions appear credible overall in its argumentation and especially in the perceived injustice he suffered. In the pamphlets of Rodig, the suffering that his family had to endure due to his absence and the subsequent stigmatization becomes particularly clear. They were barely provided with food and clothing, nor did they have permanent housing.

His first pamphlet was published in a small Publishing House in Chemnitz in 1896 and consists of 68 pages. The title is: "A case of Forbes in Saxony or How someone can gradually go mad. Experiences of J. A. Rodig in Leipzig-Lindenau, Luppenstraße 12. The net profit is intended for the unhappy Rodig's family. [transl., T. H.]"[9] In his first brochure, Rodig, a trained shoemaker, goes into detail about his origins and family circumstances and then explains how it came about that he was interned several times in prisons and institutions. One of his main concerns was (probably) the attempt to obtain an inheritance. To achieve that he even filed a lawsuit against the tax authorities. Primarily the brochure seems to have been written in order to prove himself as the rightful heir. Cornelia Brink suspects that Rodig did not write the pamphlet himself, due to the linguistic style it represents. However, this can be neither verified nor falsified, for in other pamphlets the editors admit to having either contributed as authors or explicitly refrained from interfering (Brink 2010, 173). Ann Goldberg already recognized the fundamental problem of the diagnosis "troublemaker insanity", because fighting for one's rights was pathological for this diagnosis and instrumentalized to confirm it (Goldberg 2003, 208). In addition, Rodig tried to improve his situation with the help of the brochure in order to compensate the unsuccessful efforts by the public in another way and to be able to be reinstated in his social status, according to Goldberg the act of "social alchemy" (*ibid.*, 198).

One aim of the publication was to show how easily someone could be declared "insane" and become legally incompetent as a result. From the publisher's point of view, it was described as follows: "[...] like a man who always and unceasingly fights against these 'sore points' that hit him hard, or who defends a right that is apparently indisputably due to him, can so easily be declared 'insane' – 'mad' or afflicted with the 'madness of troublemakers' by

---

9   Original title: Rodig, Johann Andreas: Ein Fall Forbes in Sachsen oder Wie Jemand nach und nach wahnsinnig werden kann. Erlebnisse des J. A. Rodig in Leipzig-Lindenau, Luppenstraße 12. Der Reinertrag ist für die unglückliche Rodig'sche Familie bestimmt. Chemnitz 1896.

court physicians or official lunatic asylum physicians, and can easily be taken to an asylum, while many private physicians and the whole environment of the unfortunate man, who are intimately involved with him, out of innermost conviction, consider the 'insane man' to be a completely healthy person! [transl., T. H.]" (Rodig 1896, 3).[10] This argument is weakened by the publishing house as they write in the following: "There are, however, cases, in which all the world considers such a man to be completely mentally clear, who, according to the proofs of psychiatrists, is not so after all; whether this is the case here, we do not want to judge. [transl., T. H.]" (*ibid.*, 4). Other than the publishing house the writers of the brochures deny the professional power of judgment of the psychiatrists.

In this first brochure, Rodig tries to prove his innocence regarding his alleged criminal offences as well as his entitlement to receive the inheritance named in the brochure. At the beginning he provides information about his origin and his life. Here, however, no major chain of argumentation regarding the normality narrative is yet to be seen (*ibid.*, 4–8). His mentioned family life is interwoven with his professional life. From 1864 to 1868 he underwent an apprenticeship as a shoemaker. Some years later, in 1877, he married Anna Emilie Walther, with whom he had four children named Hans, Linna, Alfred and Anna (*ibid.*, 6, 8, 48).[11] At first glance, he seems to live a 'regular life', according to the basic data about his profession and family – a socially expected course of life. However, the breaks in his life are made clear by the professional difficulties and the stays in the institutions and the previous convictions mentioned in the second brochure.

The topics of family, profession and social life/environment emerge explicitly in his argumentation in the second pamphlet: "Without rights in a constitutional state or to declare somebody insane is no witchcraft. Lawful injustices

---

10   Rodig, *Ein Fall Forbes*, Original: "[...] wie ein Mensch, der immer und unaufhörlich gegen diese ihn schwer treffenden 'wunden Punkte' ankämpft, oder der ein, ihm augenscheinlich unbestreitbar zuliegendes *Recht* verfechtet, gar so leicht von Gerichtsärzten oder behördlichen Irrenanstaltsärzten für 'irrsinnig' – 'verrückt' oder vom 'Querulantenwahn' befallen *erklärt* und ohne Weiteres in's Irrenhaus 'Zgebracht werden kann, während doch viele Privatärzte und die ganze Umgebung des Unglücklichen, die auf's Intimste mit ihm verkehren, aus innerster Ueberzeugung heraus den 'Geisteskrankseinsollenden' für einen völlig gesunden Menschen halten!"

11   Rodig, Johann Andreas: Rechtlos im Rechtsstaate oder irrsinnig erklären ist keine Hexerei. Rechtmässige Ungerechtigkeiten und Irrtümer dargest. von deren Opfer Johann Andreas Rodig. München/Leipzig 1897, 26; Stadtarchiv Leipzig: Krankenakte Rodig, Johann Andreas, in: Bestand Landesheil- u. Pflegeanstalt Dösen, Inventar Nr. 233/Einzelakten 18201, 1.

and errors portrayed by their victims. [transl., T. H.]" published in 1897.[12] This title represents the motivation to point out the "injustices" he experienced, namely what happened to him in a "constitutional state" on a legal basis and, in his view, made him a victim of the system. The association of "insanity" with the term "witchcraft" indicates a negative connotation. For the term "witch" is understood in contemporary terms as a form of "damage" and connection with evil or the devil. In this way, the fact that a declaration of insanity is a legal process is contradicted and the real-existing constellation is contrasted with a "supernatural effect". Deriving from the title, Rodig's argument is that he does not regard the fact of declaring someone "insane" as neither "lawless" nor a "magical" process. In German, the phrase "Das ist kein Hexenwerk"/"This is no witchcraft" is synonymous with the simplicity of an activity or its execution (Hexenwerk 2021, n.p.). With this paraphrase, Rodig and the editor deliberately discredit the state in its regulations and their handling. The focus is on the perceived arbitrariness of the state in providing for committal to an insane asylum. The second brochure concentrates more on his life and his suffering, his feeling lost and being robbed of all his rights.

The first chapter's title is "Passionpath" and focusses on his suffering. He portrays his circle of misfortunes, starting in his childhood, continuing with his apprenticeship, assistant period, and his lost apprenticeship, "The marriage brings the first blow of fate", unemployment, before eventually resulting in unjustified arrestment (*ibid.*). He also mentions the negotiation in parliament, which only decided that is was right for him to be labelled insane and there is no reason to indemnify him for his supposedly lost inheritance.[13] In this second pamphlet, he deals in detail with his various employment relationships and the search for work. He writes about his apprenticeship as a shoemaker and the years afterwards, about the fact that he had lost his father and therefore came to his position of breadwinner. Later he is forced by work to move places with his wife and children several times, facing a common problem for many people of their time.

---

12   Rodig, Johann Andreas: Rechtlos im Rechtsstaate oder irrsinnig erklären ist keine Hexerei. Rechtmässige Ungerechtigkeiten und Irrtümer dargest. von deren Opfer Johann Andreas Rodig. München; Leipzig 1897.

13   Mittheilungen über die Verhandlungen des Landtags. I. Kammer. Dresden 10. Januar 1894. Nr. 11, in: Mittheilungen über die Verhandlungen des Landtags im Königreiche Sachsen während der Jahre 1893 und 1894. I. Kammer. Dresden o. J. 73–79, here 77. And also: Mittheilungen über die Verhandlungen des Landtags. II. Kammer. Dresden 30. Januar 1894. Nr. 33, in: Mittheilungen über die Verhandlungen des Landtags im Königreiche Sachsen während der Jahre 1893 und 1894. II. Kammer. Dresden o. J. 441–446, here 445.

After he was discharged from the army, another challenge arose: "It was difficult for me to be active in my craft again, which I had not practiced for three years, but I managed to get housework for a factory again, but only for a short time. The mechanical shoe manufacturing came into swing and completely displaced the manual work, I could regard my apprenticeship almost completely as lost time and in the 25 years of my life I had to decide to start a new apprenticeship [transl., T. H.]" (Rodig 1897, 14). The hardship that emerges is that "[i]t was not possible for me to get work and starvation was the order of the day for me. [transl., T. H.]" (*ibid.*, 12). Furthermore: "I believed that the evil time was over now, and that trusting in my manpower, I would be able to feed myself. But what happened? A labour shortage occurred in the factory and numerous workers, including myself, were laid off. [transl., T. H.]" (*ibid.*, 15). Other text passages are similar. His complaining about the situation is explicit. Yet he has had problems to find work and stay employed, because new accusations were constantly brought up against him, resulting in the loss of his job over and over again at short notice. Further accusations against him are for example the insult to the Emperor's majesty or of being a member of the socialist party which was forbidden at that time. However, he also declares the accusations to be a "storm" and "strokes of fate" that overtook him and for which he could not be held responsible. The employer's side cannot be investigated at this stage, since no files on them could be found.

The third brochure titled "New revelations and publications of medical reports and court decisions of the Schumacher Johann Andreas Rodig in Leipzig, who has been declared mentally ill: truthful descriptions of an incapacitated person in the Kingdom of Saxony. [transl., T. H.]" published in 1902 has 43 pages and is an author's edition.[14] Choosing this title, Rodig obviously aims to complement the previous brochures. The expert opinions are supposed to confirm his state of health and underline the lapse of the diagnosis of "troublemaker insanity". It is essentially a collection of newspaper articles, medical certificates, official documents and reports. Documents that explain the strokes of fate that made him a troublemaker.

Several times he clarifies that he considers himself healthy and that everything else overtook him. It seems that he had no part in these so-called "blows of fate", following a statement from the second brochure as an example: "If I am bothering the readers of this writing with a short sketch of my life, please

---

14   Rodig, Johann Andreas: Neue Enthüllungen und Veröffentlichungen von ärztlichen Gutachten und gerichtlichen Beschlüssen des für geisteskrank erklärten Schumacher Johann Andreas Rodig in Leipzig: Wahrheitsgetreue Schilderungen eines Entmündigten im Königreich Sachsen. Probstheida/Leipzig 1902.

do not consider it as an outflow of megalomania, from which I might be biased. I am not aware of any greatness that could count me among the immortal. If I am nevertheless presenting my life story here, it is to show in its entirety the chain of blows of fate that have followed me up to now, from which everyone will have to draw the conclusion that my spiritual constitution must be an abnormally strong one if I have not yet lost my mind despite what I have experienced. [transl., T. H.]" (Roding 1897, 5).

In summary, it can be said that through the various aspects of the *normality narrative* – family, work, social life, health – the attempt is made to be seen as *normal* and to demonstrate a regulated life. It seems that he is trying to lead a regular life and to be employed again, to feed his family and find a stable structure. However, the various accusations do not allow him to stay in a job permanently. According to his description he experiences these accusations repeatedly and is not involved in them. He takes a passive role, feeling powerless against the events that seem beyond his control. He doubts that he might be ill and – as the brochures clearly state – he always seeks proof that he is healthy and therefore *normal*. Even in the mental hospital, according to his descriptions, he sees himself as the healthy one among the sick. His family situation is also regulated from an external view, but he cannot take care of them and they do not only have to suffer hunger, precisely because of all the accusations made against him.

The second case is about Pauline Charlotte von Süßmilch gen. Hörnig who was born on 23 January 1853 as a daughter of a Saxonian lieutenant colonel. She remained unmarried[15] and was a teacher of the French language. To what extent she was able to pursue her profession as a teacher is unknown. The job title as stated in her medical file at Thonberg Sanatorium is (dt.) "Privata", which means that she or her family had good financial resources.[16] It becomes apparent at this early stage that her case differs greatly from the previous one in a number of aspects. She wrote one pamphlet with 130 pages and there is one patient record of her containing more than 100 pages. She was in several asylums and did not deny suffering from "mental distress", in this case religious insanity: "I would like to point out that the reader of these sheets cannot make a clinical picture of me from the examples I have given myself. But perhaps it would be useful if I added that in my case mania religiosa has always developed

15   Stadtarchiv Leipzig: Krankenakte Süßmilch, Paula Charlotte von, in: Bestand 1.3.4.10.2. Heilanstalt Thonberg / Einzelakten 57–188, 9.
16   *Ibid.*, 15.

from persecution mania [transl., T. H.]."[17] In her brochure, she makes suggestions that belong within the framework of the women's movement, such as
her demand for female guards. The title is "A contribution to the question of
the training/apprenticeship of female guards in mental hospitals, based on
my insights and experiences in four Saxony mental hospitals, preceded by a
brief overview of the development history of psychiatry [transl., T. H.]."[18] She
chooses a scientific approach, using footnotes and providing a historical retro-
spect. In her pamphlet, she writes from an outside perspective, providing an
inside view of work in an asylum. She gives precise incentives for the improvement and elimination of the conditions and grievances for the institutions she
'sees' and she makes suggestions for improvement from her own experiences:
She was a wealthy woman. "Occupation distracts both from delusional ideas,
and it also re-develops paralyzed willpower and allows the proverb: 'Idleness
is the beginning of all vice' to be rightly applied to the increase of delusional
ideas and melancholy caused by inactivity. The lunatics must be taught to work
on their own recovery [transl., T. H.]."[19] Thus, in her opinion, recovery is not
possible without work. Conversely, this suggests that one cannot stay healthy
without work. Later in her pamphlet, she develops this thought even further:
"Even if the benefits of work are no longer overlooked in any institution today,
they have not become the rule. For the men there are no workshops, gardens,
parks, even if sometimes many fields of muscle work. In most of the better
institutions, however, life passes under oppressive, physical idleness, which
leaves the sick the whole day to their dreams, without providing them with
the muscle fatigue that works through night sleep. In this way, one can drive
the most reasonable person mad. While spiritual activity, which can be more
easily introduced through books, games, plays, social associations, arouses the
brain, which should be calmed, thus easily disturbs the balance between soul

---

17   Original: "Einschalten möchte ich hier, daß der Leser dieser Blätter aus den von mir selbst
      erzählten Beispielen sich kein Krankheitsbild von mir machen kann. Vielleicht ist es aber
      nützlich, wenn ich hinzufüge, daß sich bei mir mania religiosa stets aus Verfolgungswahn
      entwickelt hat." (Süßmilch-Hörnig, Ein Beitrag zu der Frage der Ausbildung der Wärterin-
      nen an Irrenanstalten, v).

18   Süßmilch-Hörnig, Pauline Charlotte von: Ein Beitrag zu der Frage der Ausbildung der
      Wärterinnen an Irrenanstalten, auf Grund meiner Einblicke und Erfahrungen in vier
      sächsischen Irrenanstalten mit Voranstellung eines kurzen Ueberblicks über die Entwick-
      lungsgeschichte der Psychiatrie. Dresden 1904.

19   Original: "Beschäftigung lenkt sowohl von Wahnideen ab, als sie auch gelähmte Willen-
      skraft wieder entwickelt und läßt sich das Sprichwort: 'Müßiggang ist aller Laster Anfang'
      mit Recht auf die durch Unbeschäftigtsein hervorgerufene Steigerung von Wahnideen
      und Melancholie anwenden. Man muß die Irren lehren, an ihrer eigenen Genesung zu
      arbeiten." (See *ibid.*, 35).

and body even more [transl., T. H.]."[20] It thus also hands over the responsibility for the recovery of the sick person, which he should strive for through work.

It can be assumed that she also held this perspective through a special status, possibly through her wealth, in the institution. Her insight into everyday life in the institution has made it clear to her how positive employment and regular daily routine had an effect on the patient. At the same time, however, she complains that such employment opportunities often do not exist. With this, she justifies her demand for the expansion of work and what was later to be named occupational therapy. In addition to the effect of work, she also includes in her presentation the condition of windows, doors and beds. One example is that she compares the window glass from her own experience and concludes that it would be better if the patient could not look out of the window because the external influences would not have a calming effect. Some of her drawings, a floor plan, in the medical file are proof of this.[21] She does not write about her family or about her social environment. She may have taken the writing of the pamphlet itself as a "job", writing altruistically for the betterment of those who came after her in the institution. She does not, however, fully conform to the normality narrative because she has accepted the diagnosis given to her. This could be an interesting gender aspect that can be pursued elsewhere. However, by positioning herself on the importance of work in the institution, she takes a stand on this aspect of work being important for a healthy life or convalescence.

7   Conclusion

The brief investigation illustrates the complexity of some aspects of the *normality narrative* – family, work, social life and environment, health. To

---

20   Original: "Wenn auch die Wohlthat der Arbeit heute in keiner Anstalt mehr verkannt wird, so ist die doch noch nicht zur Regel geworden. Für die Männer fehlen die Werkstätten, die Gärten, Parks, wenn auch manchmal etliche Felder der Muskelarbeit dienen. In den meisten der besseren Anstalten vergeht jedoch das Leben unter erdrückendem körperlichen [sic!] Müßiggang, welcher den Kranken den ganzen Tag seinen Träumen überläßt, ohne ihm die den Nachtschlaf wirkende Muskelermüdung zu verschaffen. So kann man den vernünftigsten Menschen verrückt machen. Während geistige Beschäftigung, welche durch Bücher, Spiele, Schauspiele, gesellige Vereinigungen leichter eingeführt werden kann, das Gehirn, welches beruhigt werden sollte, erregt, also leicht das Gleichgewicht zwischen Seele und Leib nur noch mehr stört." (See *ibid.*, 59).

21   Stadtarchiv Leipzig: Krankenakte Süßmilch, Paula Charlotte von, in: Bestand 1.3.4.10.2. Heilanstalt Thonberg / Einzelakten 57–188, 44.

be *normal*, means as shown, to lead or to demonstrate a regulated life that is socially accepted. The investigation shows that further analysis is necessary to get a clearer result. A reference to the narrative itself and the conditions could for example be an additional approach for the analysis. Moreover, by including subjectivation via biography, another aspect could be added to refine the analysis.

In the two briefly examined cases from the margins of society, Pauline Charlotte Süßmilch gen. Hörnig seems to stand above the things, even though she is actually affected by them. This contrasts with the case of Johann Andreas Rodig. He has an inner perspective as being concerned. Süßmilch does not write about her profession, because she may not have worked much as a woman, or because of her wealth. This may also be the reason, why she has taken an observational perspective. She is a well-educated woman. He seems to have received less education recognizable by his profession. In addition, their socioeconomic status is independent and dependent. Also, Rodig is affected by industrialisation – the exercise of his profession is only possible in a modified form. It should be noted that these two cases are contrary to each other and clearly underline their positions in society and their dependence on socioeconomic status. She seems to have a regular routine inside the institution and he tries to lead a regular life outside the institution. But none of them has a fully accepted life situation. By acknowledging the diagnosis given to her, she takes a different position, as she seems to have come to terms with her life circumstances and does not suffer, at least she does not narrate her suffering. Rodig stands in contrast to this, as he tries to reduce his suffering, even though the three publications show that he tries to lead a regular life despite all adversities. He denies being ill and classifies himself as normal, but she does not doubt nor does she discuss it. It can be assumed that there are different kinds of *normalities* to be observed here. These need to be defined more precisely in a further analysis.

In my analysis, I use the inside perspective from the pamphlets and the outside perspective from the medical records. As a result, I aim to show how a separated member of society regains or tries to regain his position as an accepted subject of society. Work is shown here to be an important aspect that corresponds to a healthy or normal way of life. At this point, as the examples of Süßmilch and Rodig make clear, work can be thought of from two perspectives: firstly, work establishes a socially accepted norm of a healthy subject; equally, secondly, from another perspective, it shows that work verifies a healthy regulated lifestyle. The importance of this aspect is addressed and recognised by Süßmilch. This form of therapy was later incorporated into general therapy, thus underlining her forward-looking view. It can be concluded by this that other aspects can be taken from the brochures that could prove useful for therapies or their development beyond the normality narrative. The brochure provides insights into their lives and into the personal feelings of those affected, which a medical record as a source cannot do. This first time ever event of writing brochures is a form of self-empowerment, which today is possibly in its continuation the self-help group, which is also a form of self-empowerment. It may have contributed to that practice in therapy.

Nobody has investigated the pamphlets with the point of view of subjectivation or self-making before. The argumentation and their behaviour can be explained in the context of interaction in societies. What happened to the self of labelled persons excluded by society? These cases show what it means to be excluded from your social field and open up for rethinking our sensitivity in dealing with and our relations to others and our behaviour.

References

Bernet, Brigitta. 2007. "Der bürgerliche Tod: Entmündigungsangst, Psychiatriekritik und die Krise des liberalen Subjektentwurfs um 1900." In *Zwang zur Ordnung. Psychiatrie im Kanton Zürich, 1870–1970*, edited by Brigitta Bernet, Marietta Meier, Roswitha Dubach, and Urs Germann, 117–153. Zürich: Chronos Verlag.

Brink, Cornelia. 2002. "'Nicht mehr normal und noch nicht geisteskrank ...': Über psychopathologische Grenzfälle im Kaiserreich." *WerkstattGeschichte* 33: 22–44.

Brink, Cornelia. 2010. *Grenzen der Anstalt: Psychiatrie und Gesellschaft in Deutschland 1860–1980. Moderne Zeit. Neue Forschungen zur Gesellschafts- und Kulturgeschichte des 19. und 20. Jahrhunderts*, vol. 20. Göttingen: Wallstein Verlag.

Canguilhem, Georges. 1974. *Das Normale und das Pathologische*. München: Matthes und Seitz.

Etzemüller, Thomas. 2012. *Biographien: Lesen – erforschen – erzählen*. Frankfurt/Main: Campus.

Fangerau, Heiner, and Karen Nolte, eds. 2006. *"Moderne" Anstaltspsychiatrie im 19. und 20. Jahrhundert – Legitimation und Kritik. Medizin, Gesellschaft und Geschichte*. Jahrbuch des Instituts für Geschichte der Medizin der Robert Bosch Stiftung, vol. 26. Stuttgart.

Fludernik, Monika, and Marie-Laure Ryan. 2020. "Factual Narrative: An Introduction." In *Narrative Factuality. A Handbook*, edited by Monika Fludernik and Marie-Laure Ryan, 1–28. Jannidis, Fotis, Gerhard Lauer, Matías Martínes, and Simone Winko, eds. *Revisionen. Grundbegriffe der Literaturtheorie*, vol. 6. Berlin/Boston: De Gruyter.

Gemoll, Wilhelm. 1991. *Griechisch-Deutsches Schul- und Handwörterbuch*. München: G. Freytag Verlag.

Goldberg, Ann. 2003. "A Reinvented Public: 'Lunatics' Rights' and Bourgeois Populism in the Kaiserreich." In *Psychiatrie im 19. Jahrhundert. Forschungen zur Geschichte von psychiatrischen Institutionen, Debatten und Praktiken im deutschen Sprachraum*, edited by Eric J. Engstrom and Volker Roelcke, 189–219. Medizinische Forschung, vol. 13. Mainz.

Hahn, Alois. 1987. "Identität und Selbstthematisierung." In *Selbstthematisierung und Selbstzeugnis: Bekenntnis und Geständnis*, edited by Alois Hahn and Volker Kapp, 9–24. Frankfurt/Main: Suhrkamp.

Heiligenthal, Peter, ed. 1985. *Denkwürdigkeiten eines Nervenkranken by Daniel Paul Schreber*. Frankfurt/Main.

Hoffmann-Richter, Ulrike. "Das Verschwinden der Biographie in der Krankenge-schichte. Eine biographische Skizze." *Bios. Zeitschrift für Biographieforschung und Oral History* 8, no. 2 (1995): 204–222.

Hofmann, Hasso, and Wolfgang H. Schrader. 1984. "Norm." In *Historisches Wörterbuch der Philosophie*, edited by Joachim Ritter and Karlfried Gründer, vol. 6: 906–920. Basel: Verlag Scheidegger and Spiess.

Kudlien, Fridolf, and Henning H. Ritter. 1984. "Normal, Normalität." In *Historisches Wörterbuch der Philosophie*, edited by Joachim Ritter and Karlfried Gründer, vol. 6: 920–928. Basel: Verlag Scheidegger and Spiess.

Lothane, Henry Zvi. 1992. In *Defense of Schreber: Soul Murder and Psychiatry*. Hillsdale, Routledge.

Nolte, Karen. "Querulantenwahnsinn – 'Eigensinn' oder 'Irrsinn'?" In *"Moderne" Anstaltspsychiatrie im 19. und 20. Jahrhundert – Legitimation und Kritik*, edited by Heiner Fangerau and Karen Nolte, vol. 26: 395–411. *Medicine, Society and History: Yearbook of the Institute for the History of Medicine of the Robert Bosch Foundation*. Stuttgart, 2006.

Santner, Eric L. 1996. *My Own Private Germany: Daniel Paul Schreber's Secret History of Modernity*. New Jersey: Princeton University Press.

Schmiedebach, Heinz-Peter. "Eine 'antipsychiatrische Bewegung' um die Jahrhundertwende." In *Medizinkritische Bewegungen im Deutschen Reich (ca. 1870–ca. 1933)*, edited by Martin Dinges and Vincent Barras, vol. 9, 127–161. *Medicine, Society and History: Yearbook of the Institute for the History of Medicine of the Robert Bosch Foundation*. Stuttgart, 1996.

Schmuhl, Hans-Walter. "Experten in eigener Sache: Der Beitrag psychiatrischer Patienten zur 'Irrenrechtsreform' im 19. und frühen 20. Jahrhundert." *Sozialpsychiatrische Information* 39, no. 3 (2009): 7–9.

Schwoch, Rebecca, and Heinz-Peter Schmiedebach. "Querulantenwahnsinn, Psychiatriekritik und Öffentlichkeit um 1900." *Medizinhistorisches Journal* 42, no. 1 (2007): 30–60.

Steinberg, Holger. "Paul Flechsig (1847–1929) – ein Hirnforscher als Psychiater." In *200 Jahre Psychiatrie an der Universität Leipzig: Personen und Konzepte*, edited by Matthias C. Angermeyer and Holger Steinberg, 81–120. Heidelberg, 2005.

Tölle, Rainer. 1987. "Die Krankengeschichte in der Psychiatrie." In *Biographie und Psychologie*, edited by Gerd Jüttemann and Hans Thomae, 36–47. Berlin: Springer.

Wolters, Christine, Christof Beyer, and Brigitte Lohff. 2013. "Abweichung und Normalität als Problem der Psychiatrie im 20. Jahrhundert." In *Abweichung und Normalität. Psychiatrie in Deutschland vom Kaiserreich bis zur Deutschen Einheit*, edited by Christine Wolters et al., 9–23. Bielefeld: Transcript.

Online Literature

Crane, Gregory R. "Perseus Digital Library (Tufts University)." http://www.perseus.tufts.edu/hopper/morph?l=dikaiotath&la=greek#lexicon (accessed October 28, 2020).

Fludernik, Monika. "Research Program of the Research Training Group 'Factual and Fictional Narrative. Differences, Interferences and Congruencies in Narratological Perspective'." Online at: http://www.grk-erzaehlen.uni-freiburg.de/wp-content/uploads/2014/05/grk1767-forschung.pdf (accessed August 24, 2020); and https://www.grk-erzaehlen.uni-freiburg.de/english-summary/ (accessed September 22, 2020).

"Hexenwerk." In Berlin-Brandenburgische Akademie der Wissenschaften: Digitales Wörterbuch der Deutschen Sprache. Online at: https://www.dwds.de/wb/Hexenwerk (accessed April 24, 2021).

Sources

Beyer, Bernhard. 1912. "Die Bestrebungen zur Reform des Irrenwesens. Material zu einem Reichs-Irrengesetz. Für Laien und Ärzte." *Psychiatrisch-Neurologische Wochenschrift*, Ergänzungsband. Halle/Saale.

Kirchenheim, Arthur von, and Heinrich Reinartz. 1895. Zur Reform des Irrenrechts. Elf Leitsätze zur Besserung der Irrenfürsorge und Beseitigung des Entmündigungsunfugs im Auftrage einer am 21. November 1894 in Göttingen zusammengetretenen Vereinigung mit Begründung herausgegeben von Professor Dr. von Kirchenheim – Heidelberg und Rechtsanwalt Dr. Reinartz – Düsseldorf. Barmen.

Krumbiegel, Friedrich Wilhelm. 1893. Gesund in's Irrenhaus! Prozesse des Kohlenspediteurs F. W. Krumbiegel in Zwickau, Sachsen. Ein Beitrag zur Beleuchtung der sächsischen Gerichtspflege. Zwickau.

Mittheilungen über die Verhandlungen des Landtags. I. Kammer. 1894. Dresden 10. Januar. Nr. 11. In Mittheilungen über die Verhandlungen des Landtags im Königreiche Sachsen während der Jahre 1893 und 1894. I. Kammer. Dresden. 73–79.

Mittheilungen über die Verhandlungen des Landtags. II. Kammer. 1894. Dresden 30. Januar. Nr. 33. In Mittheilungen über die Verhandlungen des Landtags im Königreiche Sachsen während der Jahre 1893 und 1894. II. Kammer. Dresden. 441–446.

Rodig, Johann Andreas. 1896. Ein Fall Forbes in Sachsen oder Wie Jemand nach und nach wahnsinnig werden kann. Erlebnisse des J. A. Rodig in Leipzig-Lindenau, Luppenstraße 12. Der Reinertrag ist für die unglückliche Rodig'sche Familie bestimmt. Chemnitz.

Rodig, Johann Andreas. 1897. Rechtlos im Rechtsstaate oder irrsinnig erklären ist keine Hexerei. Rechtmässige Ungerechtigkeiten und Irrtümer dargest. von deren Opfer Johann Andreas Rodig. München/Leipzig.

Rodig, Johann Andreas. 1902. Neue Enthüllungen und Veröffentlichungen von ärztlichen Gutachten und gerichtlichen Beschlüssen des für geisteskrank erklärten Schumacher Johann Andreas Rodig in Leipzig: Wahrheitsgetreue Schilderungen eines Entmündigten im Königreich Sachsen. Probstheida/Leipzig.

Schreber, Daniel Paul. 1973. Bürgerliche Wahnwelt um Neunzehnhundert. Denkwürdigkeiten eines Nervenkranken von Daniel Paul Schreber (Der Fall Schreber 1). Wiesbaden.

Süßmilch-Hörnig, Pauline Charlotte von. 1904. Ein Beitrag zu der Frage der Ausbildung der Wärterinnen an Irrenanstalten, auf Grund meiner Einblicke und Erfahrungen in vier sächsischen Irrenanstalten mit Voranstellung eines kurzen Ueberblicks über die Entwicklungsgeschichte der Psychiatrie. Dresden.

Stadtarchiv Leipzig. Krankenakte Rodig, Johann Andreas. Bestand Landesheil- u. Pflegeanstalt Dösen, Inventar Nr. 233/Einzelakten 18201.

Stadtarchiv Leipzig. Krankenakte Süßmilch, Paula Charlotte von. Bestand 1.3.4.10.2. Heilanstalt Thonberg / Einzelakten 57–188.

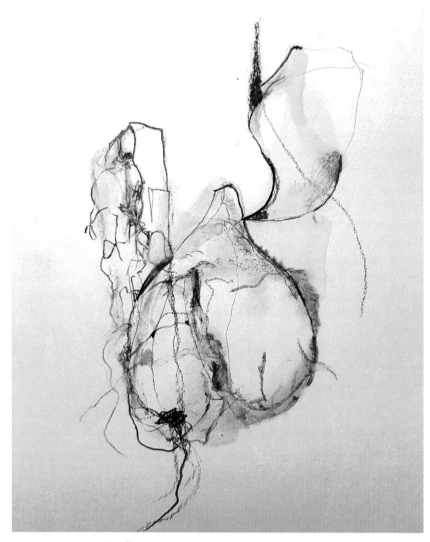

FIGURE 8.1   Marta Wandt

CHAPTER 9

"The Small Point through which Time Passes" – Art and Artistic Practices in Former Mental Healthcare Institutions

Hedvig Mårdh

Abstract

Artistic practices are increasingly used by and integrated into the management of cultural heritage. In the chapter the author explores the associations made between mental health and artistic creativity, as well as the inclusion of contemporary art and artistic practices in sites with a complex history, such as former psychiatric hospitals. The article is based on a research project about the redevelopment of Ulleråker, a former psychiatric hospital in Sweden. Photographic practices in abandoned sites, patients' art, artistic interventions in the Museum of Medical History, as well as the pre-study work by artist Camille Norment and the public artwork by Lies-Marie Hoffman, are discussed in relation to heritage management and the concept of third-time. The article shows how artistic practices in Ulleråker and similar sites, such as Beckomberga and Lillhagen, have in different ways helped to negotiate time as well as complex histories, when the sites are deinstitutionalised and turned into offices and housing.

Keywords

cultural heritage – patient art – public art – third-time – Ulleråker

1   Introduction

Art and artistic practices are increasingly used by and integrated in city development, often acting as a place-marketing tool in a creative city agenda. Moreover, art has become an integral part of the management and understanding of complex heritage sites such as abandoned psychiatric hospitals and, the in many cases conflicting histories connected to these sites (e.g., Popescu and Schult 2020; Rodéhn and Mårdh 2021, 30; Mårdh 2021, 75–79).

There are numerous examples where municipalities and property developers commission art works and invite artistic practices by offering funding for project and studios, purposefully moving artists into these sites. Our study of Ulleråker and other similar sites shows that associations made between mental health and artistic creativity have been consciously maintained, used, and mediated when former psychiatric hospitals are transformed into residential areas. The conscious introduction of art is often motivated and supported by a pragmatic understanding of art's societal impact, where art is used to sustain or co-produce "a certain notion of history, progress, and development" (Hantelmann 2010). However, I agree with the historian of ideas Klas Grinell that this kind of instrumental view of art does not necessarily exclude that art's own value is recognised by the actors involved in the process (Grinell 2019, 3).

One of the qualities of artistic practice, in relation to heritage, is that it can support narratives that challenge time as a linear succession of instants. I suggest that art could be seen as a *third-time tool* in relation to the heritage of psychiatry. Third-time is a concept established by Paul Ricoeur who developed his ideas about the concept of time throughout his long academic career (Ricoeur 1980; Malan 2017). Third-time tools, for example archives, documents and traces, mediate between *subjective*, lived time and *objective* time, creating *cultural time* (Fornäs 2016, 5215). Inspired by Ricoeur's understanding of time and Johan Fornäs (2016) exploration of third-time tools I will look closer at art and artistic practice in relation to the heritage of psychiatry. Artists have for a long time been key narrators of history, working alongside traditional institutions to remember, glorify and mourn the past. Today, we see how some of these monuments are being torn down, as people question their ideological meaning and authority over history. Political and social movements, such as Black Lives Matter, have shown that public art can be used, not only to glorify but also to suppress past and present narratives. This calls for awareness also among contemporary artists, not the least since they are increasingly working in parallel with cultural economy planning, community-based art programs and place-marketing in sites with a complex history. Ideally art can help provide diverse and nuanced interpretations of the past in such contexts. However, we need better insights into how art and artists can do this and how art can contribute to a sustainable use and reuse of historic sites such as former psychiatric hospitals.

The chapter starts by considering the concept of time in relation to public art, it then focuses on the historical relation between mental health and art, and how patients' art works have been made available to the public as part of a heritage process. It then continues by discussing different types of visual and spatial explorations of former hospitals – photography in relation to urban exploration, patients' art and contemporary art, which in different ways can help mediate the complex cultural heritage and narrative on site.

2   Clarifying Time in Former Psychiatric Hospitals

This study is based on the research project *From psychiatric hospital to condominium – urban development and cultural heritage* (Formas 2019-00589). The project focuses on the redevelopment of Ulleråker, a former psychiatric hospital in Sweden. Being an art historian focusing on cultural heritage, museums, and public art I am interested in how the understandings and attitudes towards the past shape the decisions made concerning art, but also how visual expressions and "material existence" can help us relate to and understand the past. This attitude is inspired by Michel Foucault, who to a large extent was a visual historian who encompassed the spaces of the past, "A period only let some things be seen and not others. [...] And this visual thought is rooted in a specific sort of 'material existence' – the spaces in which it is exercised (such as hospital, prison, museum, or home) ..." (Rajchman 1988, 92). Further I've been inspired by Paul Ricoeur's understanding of time and Johan Fornäs (2016) exploration of third-time tools, and I will look closer at art and artistic practice in relation to narratives and the heritage of psychiatry. The material analysed includes art works, documentation of artistic practices, exhibition documentation and official document such as the art program for Ulleråker (Uppsala kommun 2017). Comparisons are made with similar former hospitals in Sweden, such as Beckomberga in Bromma, Stockholm, and Lillhagen in Gothenburg.

Ulleråker had been the site of a hospital since the 1810s, and until the 1990s it was the permanent or temporary home of thousands of individuals, patients, and staff. It housed about 1300 patients when it was at maximum capacity. On site, there is a cemetery with 1290 individual graves, most of them unmarked patients' graves. Ulleråker is situated in Uppsala, where Michel Foucault wrote most of what would become his doctoral thesis *Histoire de la folie à l'âge Classique, folie et déraison* (1961). Ulleråker shares many of the characteristics of the asylums described by Foucault, however, since the psychiatric care has moved from the site, another layer is being added. Today, parts of Ulleråker have been turned into housing while other buildings are empty, waiting for demolition or reuse, when 7–8.000 more apartments are built. At the moment it is primarily the spatial form that embodies and represents the past on site, there are few traces of the societal practices of the displaced people who lived and worked in the hospital. Researchers Graham Moon, Robin Kearns and Alun Joseph (2015) show that when making the choice of what to preserve or what to destroy in post-asylum landscapes such as Ulleråker, there is a process of "strategic forgetting and selective remembrance".

> ... selective remembrance serves as a counterpoint to the silences of strategic forgetting and represents an important dimension of the agency exercised by stakeholders in the re-development process. These complementary concepts interrogate the creative tension between the retention of positive memories of the asylum and the simultaneous obscuring of more negative aspects of that past. (Moon, Kearns, and Joseph 2015, 26)

Psychiatric hospitals have been closed and demolished or redeveloped across the globe since the 1980s. They are often situated on attractive plots of land, and city authorities now face the challenge of integrating these former *heterotopias of deviation*, to refer to Foucault's concept, into the urban sprawl (Foucault 1986, 22). One might even claim that "asylum adaptation has become mainstream [and] part of 'normal' society" (Franklin 2010). When former psychiatric hospitals are redeveloped there is a clear break in the use of the site. How to relate to the past and use it for the present can be difficult and time can be "a visible and tangible problem" as the historian François Hartog describes the situation in Berlin after 1989 (Hartog 2015, 10). He suggests that the relation to time must be clarified before decisions and actions, such as redevelopment, are taken.

> What should the relations with the past be, or rather with pasts in the plural, but also, and no less importantly, with the future? Not forgetting the present, while also avoiding the other extreme, that of being blind to anything beyond it. In other words: how to inhabit the present, in the most literal sense? What should be destroyed, preserved, reconstructed, or built, and how? For any decisions and actions to be taken, relations to time had first to be clarified. (Hartog 2015, 10)

In a former psychiatric hospital time can be problematic. It is many-layered, overlapping, and difficult to understand, however fragments, signs, and traces that can help a present-day visitor or resident to grasp the time that has passed. Thus, our experience of time is intimately linked to the visual, to space and our experience of space, which is also an important aspect of public art. I would argue that artwork, and artistic practices can be regarded a communication practice creating an "intersubjectively shared or *cultural time*", especially if the art is site-specific and relational (Fornäs 2016, 5219). Art becomes a mode of localization and inhabiting (Fornäs 2016:5219–20) – same as the process of collecting, mapping, naming, landscaping and architecture (discussed in this anthology by Baur, pp. 13 and Rodéhn, pp. 122). However, the tools of third-time are not constant. As all media they change over time and art is no exception. Monuments of the past and contemporary art can affect people's understanding of time in different ways.

For us to understand the past, we tend to create narratives. This is also happening when art is created for and in relation to a heritage site. However, the artist can approach the narrative in different ways. In the article "Narrative Time" (1980), Paul Ricoeur present three different approaches to time: firstly, time as that "in which events take place". In this sense, it has a "datable, public, and measurable nature" (1980, 170). This could be materialised by the artists in a work depicting a specific event, presented with a date, a name or a location that help the public interpret the work. Secondly, the work can emphasise "the weight of the past and, even more, in terms of the power of recovering the 'extension' between birth and death in the work of repetition" (1980, 171). This approach is more thematic and can help the public to understand what could be learned from the past, how history repeats itself. It could be a memorial about a war or the holocaust that talks about loss, suffering or crimes committed. Thirdly, Ricoeur speaks about "the plot" which he defines as "the intelligible whole that governs a succession of events in any story" (1980, 171). This would result in an artwork that tells a story; it could be the story of the life of an individual or a specific site, a story that moves beyond the anecdotic surface of the story. If the goal is to make history relatable, "the plot" might be effective, however, Ricoeur argues that most historians "have a poor concept of 'event' – and even of 'narrative'; instead, they consider history to be an explanatory endeavour that has severed its ties with storytelling" (1980, 171). Even if the remembrance that artists and artworks 'do' has to be a selective remembrance, art can be consciously used to present complex or contradictory narratives. Moreover, art as a third-time tool can help challenge destruction of the site or the displacement of peoples resulting from the change of use and redevelopment.

3   Art, Creativity, and the Psychiatric Institution

Art and creativity have played important roles in psychiatric hospitals, both as occupation, therapy and ornamentation. In addition to the patients who have chosen to be creative on their own accord, most hospitals have offered some form of art or craft as therapeutic or recreational activities. The objects made have sometimes been sold to members of staff or to the public. However, it is important to recognise that the relation between art and mental health is complex and that many artists find it difficult to create art when being unwell and in care.

The popularised idea of a close link between the artist's creativity, originality and psychiatric diagnosis was reinforced by the nineteenth-century Romantic cult of the artist as a visionary, and to stand outside mainstream society is still a key element in how 'the artist' is popularly portrayed. The psychiatric institution has for a long time been seen as the irrefutable proof that someone is 'outside' society and the established art world. This romanticised alienation from society, balancing between acceptance and rejection, between health and sickness is both sought-after and shunned (Maclagan 2012, 11). Some artists are intimately linked to mental distress in the public mind. Swedish examples are Carl Fredrik Hill and Sigrid Hjertén. Internationally well-known artists include Vincent van Gogh, Francisco de Goya and Edvard Munch. While we find some of our most famous artists in this group, there is also a common idea in the art world that the outsider should not be interested in being known, accepted, or making a living from their creative work (Chilvers and Glaves-Smith 2015). Unfortunately, the situation for many collections of patients' art is that they are inadequately cared for and threatened by neglect. This is unfortunate, in addition to being valuable works of art, they are invaluable historical documents that need our attention and care.

Several different terms have been used to describe art associated with mental distress – *l'art brut*, *outsider art* or *patient art*. While *outsider* and similar concepts can be considered problematic and reproduce a stereotypical image of the role of the artists and people suffering from mental distress it has also helped contribute to a re-evaluation and increased appreciation of creative individuals. By collecting, exhibiting, and writing about art created in this context, artists might receive recognition and appreciation, although for most of these artists recognition might be posthumous or even anonymous. Apart from a few more well-known artists, such as those mentioned and those who had an established career outside the hospital, there is little known about patient art, and little has been saved for the future. The collections of patient's art works that do exist have usually been brought together by staff, generally in prominent positions, who have collected them at work or with the help of colleagues. Many of these collections are currently part of collections at museums of medical history or psychiatry. The initial purpose of these collections was often associated with diagnostics, education, or research in the field of psychopathology. The interest to collect and show patients' art works grew after the German psychiatrist Hans Prinzhorn published his book

Bildnerei der Geisteskranken (1922). The collection he initiated, *Sammlung Prinzhorn* in Heidelberg, has grown since, and today it contains about 20,000 objects. However, already in 1915, Bror Gadelius, a Swedish professor at Karolinska Institutet in Stockholm published the article, "Om sinnessjukdom, diktning och skapande konst" (On Mental Illness, Poetry and Creative Art, translation mine), covering the subject. Gadelius also created a large collection of art, including both anonymous and well-known Swedish artists such as Carl Fredrik Hill and Ernst Josephson.

In Europe, there are many examples of professionally run art galleries directly linked to psychiatric hospitals, for example, Bethlem gallery (UK), The House of Artists (Austria) and Museum Ovartaci (Denmark). Some of these galleries collaborate with care facilities or museums on site. These galleries usually exhibit patients' art or artists who work with relevant themes, such as war-related trauma or historical understandings of the human body. Art with connections to psychiatric hospitals has undoubtedly become more accessible to Swedish audiences after the closures. Some art has been documented and exhibited online by museums such as Medicinhistoriska samlingen at Kulturen, Lund and Psykiatriska museet, Västervik. There are also initiatives such as the *Mad Heritage & Contemporary Art*, which recognise former patients as important actors in managing the cultural heritage of psychiatry (Mad Heritage & Contemporary Art, 2020). Art has generally become more accessible on site when closed hospitals are opened to the public. Here, patients' art can often still be found on site, on walls and forgotten in storages. When the tunnels underneath Beckomberga and Lillhagen were threatened with demolition or renovation, respectively, a focus was placed on the wall paintings and artworks that might be destroyed in the process. (Narratives from Lillhagen are further discussed in Punzi and Lindbom's text in this anthology.) These paintings at Beckomberga and Lillhagen had previously only been available for and seen by a selection of staff and patients. The threat of their removal sparked different initiatives, the paintings were shown to the public and documented. Public *finissages* (final shows) were organised in Beckomberga (2017) and Lillhagen (2018). In the media, the paintings were described as "eerie" and "unusual" (SVT, Anders Nordqvist 2017). Today, most of the paintings at Beckomberga have been destroyed and those at Lillhagen are still under threat. The critic Boel Ulfsdotter suggested in her article in *Göteborgs Posten* that the paintings have not been better protected because, "the patients' paintings are included in the more sordid chapters of the city's narrative" (Translation mine, Ulfsdotter 2018–04–19). Although the sordidness and darkness of these formerly closed tunnels is also what seems to attract and invite attention from the public.

4   Aesthetics and the Sigh of Relief

When these hospitals are turned into residential areas they go through a period where they are emptied of people and the buildings exist in a state of neglect. It seems as if their emptiness and run-down state is precisely what attracts numerous photographers, film makers, artists, and urban explorers. The photographer and social historian Mark Davis has documented former asylums from the Victorian era, such as West Riding Pauper Lunatic Asylum in Meston, England. In 2014, he published the book *Asylum – Inside the Pauper Lunatic Asylums*. He finds that the photographs from these sites "take us to a world far removed from our own where we can justifiably breathe a sigh of relief and be thankful that the days of possibility of incarceration in a lunatic asylum are over" (Davis 2014, 7). The photographs in Davis' books but also other similar photographs, such as those taken by the Swedish author Jan Jörnmark, convey a feeling of a parallel reality, a reality that probably most consumers of the photographs are happy to escape, while they at the same time can be tempting to visit from your armchair or as tourists.

Like Mark Davis, the economic historian Jan Jörnmark has documented sites in this in-between state, between closing down and transformation. His photographs show abandoned industries, amusement parks and psychiatric hospitals, and together with his TV-shows, exhibitions, and books, like *Övergivna platser* (2007, 2008), they have contributed to an increased interest in urban exploration in Sweden. Jörnmark helped start the Facebook-group *Övergivna platser* (Abandoned sites) which has over 300.000 members (Övergivna platser 2021). Abandoned psychiatric hospitals are among the most popular sites, repeatedly documented and posted in the group. Jörnmark has documented several hospitals in his published books, for example Ulleråker and Sidsjöns hospital, which he photographed before it was converted into a residential area (Övergivna platser två 2008). The description of Sidsjön is integrated with a description of former care, medication, and the closing of the hospitals. The photographs show a run-down site with graffiti and old bathtubs, resembling the documentation of numerous similar sites.

The sites have a strong creative potential in their abandoned state, and generate new visits, photographs, and stories. The practice of photography creates an intimacy and closeness with the abandoned sites, which in other case would be hidden and forgotten during this period of transition (Pétursdóttir and Olsen 2014). Moreover, the photographs taken can be considered as vital documentation of these sites and can add to the occasionally lacking documentation done by the heritage sector, for example museums or The National Heritage Board. However, the run-down state of the sites is not what the patients or staff experienced when living and working there, and therefore they create only weak connections to any memories and say little of the life lived and experienced in these sites. They show fragments from earlier times in spaces that previously have been closed for visitors. Moreover, these photographs of abandoned hospitals are usually left to communicate on their own devices, there is little text accompanying them. Because of this lack of information, the narratives that the photographs generate are often subject to generalisations, presumptions, and the imagination of the spectator. Occasionally these expectations and assumptions "spill over" into the materiality of the sites themselves. They are staged with props to feed into feelings of alienation, dread, and horror.

To document and make these sites visible is important. What these photographs do best is perhaps that they give the sites a renewed aesthetical value, often aiming at capturing the beauty of decay and impermanence. However, the aesthetical and persuasive power of the photographs can also be understood as romanticising, corrupting the materiality of the site as well as being politically problematic (Pusca 2014, 35). Still, if the representations of the sites keep emphasising the strangeness and eeriness of the sites, they tend to lock in on stereotypical representations of mental distress and psychiatric care mediated in films, literature and media. It is all too easy to forget that these sites never looked like this when being a place for treatment. They were part of people's everyday life, good and bad, and we need imagery that leaves us with more than a feeling of alienation and a sigh of relief.

The process behind different types of representation of mental distress and psychiatric care has been investigated by the researcher in media and cultural studies, Simon Cross, in his book *Mediating Madness: Mental Distress and Cultural Representation* (2010). Cross describes how hospitals and illnesses are visualised and mediated in TV and film, and how visual stereotypes change over time. Patients are often mediated as "mad, bad and dangerous to know" (Cross 2004, 199). The difference between sickness and health, calm patients and potentially violent ones is constructed in the visual material he has examined. It is, according to these mediations of patients possible to *see* who is "mad" and the patient's inner struggles are clearly visible on the outside. The idea that it would be possible to identify who is sick through visual observation was established during the second half of the nineteenth century when photography was introduced into medical practice (Brookes 2011, 30). Cross emphasises that we should try to avoid stereotypical representations of madness, many of them deriving from these early photographs, but also film and literature, since this would help change attitudes. Other stereotypes come from broader cultural assumptions. Hoffman and Hansen's (2017) study of depression memoirs shows that men often describe how they turn their depression "into creative fire", while women suffering from depression portray themselves as needy and "victims of a chemical flaw" (Hoffman and Hansen 2017, 295). There are some risks if the narratives told only fall into these two gendered categories. As Hoffman and Hansen conclude "memoirs' themes of neediness and uncreativity succeed in becoming absorbed into readers' selves in this way, the selves which subsume them may be more likely to experience stereotypes of psychiatric inability than to realise creative ability" (2017, 295). Instead, Cross suggests, we should look for representations that are more open and varied (Cross 2004, 213). Davis and Jörnmark help document a period of transition, that in many cases can go on for decades. Their photographs make these sites visible and set people's imagination in motion but often they also feed into the stereotypes mentioned. If we are looking to convey about the lives lived in these complex sites, we need a variation of visual and spatial representations.

5   Contemporary Art – Relational and Site-Specific

In 1937, the Swedish parliament decided that 1% of the state budget for building should be set aside for public art. Many municipalities and regions also follow this principle. This has given public art a prominent position in building and planning projects all over Sweden. Public art can play an important role in assisting the transformation of former hospitals being turned into residential areas. Research shows that art and artistic practises increasingly help architects and urban developers in the planning process (Metzger 2010). Artists are also contributing by focusing on aspects such as ecological, economic, social, and cultural sustainability (Bennett, Reid, and Petocz 2014). In relation to former psychiatric hospitals, artistic practices have also helped negotiate the complex history of a site. The art program for Ulleråker *KUR – Konst Ulleråker – Farvatten – droppa, forsa, stänk* ("KUR - Art Ulleråker – Waters – drip, gush, splash", translation mine) has been actively integrated in the planning process since 2017. In the program, two politicians, one project manager, one art consultant and one museum director express their expectations on art and artistic practices. Among other things, they hope that art will help preserve the historical value of the area, represent diversity and a connection between past and present, and tell the stories of the patients – both the positive and the negative. Moreover, they want art to contribute to the attraction and sustainability of the new residential area, as well as strengthen the identity of the area, make the new residents and visitors reflect on their lives and the complexity of contemporary life, discuss mental health and functionality (Magnusson and Uppsala kommun 2017). The municipality encourage artists to choose Uller-åker by offering stipends and affordable workspaces. Moreover, they support exhibitions and commission public art works. Since 2020, ambitious yearly exhibitions have been organised by Konstfrämjandet (People's Movement for Art Promotion), establishing Ulleråker as a site for art. So far, these exhibitions have all related to the site and its history in different ways. The art critic Nils Forsberg (2022) found that the exhibition "*Öppna* dörrar" (Open Doors) made the concept of heterotopia more tangible – "the soul of the site was further enhanced, the past and present are connected by a suggested history of mad-ness" (authors translation "platsens själ förhöjs ytterligare, forntid och nutid binds samman av en antydd vansinnets historia").

Public art is generally labelled as *permanent* or *temporary*, for example, when realised as an event or process. However, the division is complicated by the fact that a temporary project can live on after its lifetime, as a memory, story, documentation, fragment, or inspiration. In addition, artworks labelled as per-manent have symbolic lives and change as there are shifts in context or the historical discourses evolve. Changes that configure our view and understand-ing of them (González-Sancho and Eeg-Tverbakk 2018, 11). Because of these complexities, we find that the division between permanent and temporary is less helpful when understanding the narrative function of art; rather, it tells us about the ownership and management of art works. In addition, the ques-tion of permanence is constantly challenged in these former hospital sites, as they seem to exist in a state of perpetual transformation. Materiality becomes evasive – as it continuously responds to changes in treatments, attitudes and resources related to the care and attitudes towards patients. Buildings, roads, and gardens are torn down or rebuilt to fit changed needs. I would suggest that the most productive concepts that help us understand contemporary art in relation to these sites would be *site-specific* and *relational*, but also the concept introduced earlier, art as a *third time tool*.

Site-specific art and relational art, especially when used in combination, offers several opportunities to address the heritage of complex sites. Site-specific art is designed for a particular location and establishes a relationship with this location. It opposes the modernist "white cube" where the artwork is deliberately taken out of context. Instead, it directly relates to the site, creating a spatio-temporal connection and often it addresses social and politi-cal conditions on site. The site-specific artwork derives its meaning from the site and most often the connection is with the history of the site: "The artist who sets out to produce work destined for public space or the public sphere must embark on a process of analysis and reading of the specific context he wishes to address, its contingency and temporality" (González-Sancho and Eeg-Tverbakk 2018, 13). The term is often used in connection to public art or landscape art such as the *Spiral Jetty* (1970) by Robert Smithson in Great Salt Lake, Utah.

The French art critic Nicolas Bourriaud defined the term *relational aesthetics* as: "an art taking as its theoretical horizon the realm of human interactions and its social context, rather than the assertion of an independent and *private* symbolic space" (Bourriaud 2002, 14). Artists are seen as facilitators rather than makers and the artist's practice focuses on meeting people, interactivity and problem-solving. Relational aesthetics can be seen as social work based in artistic practice: "The artist, in this sense, gives audiences access to power and the means to change the world" (Tate, undated). One example of a site-specific, relational art project funded according to the principle of 1%, is *1% love and devotion* carried out at Ulleråker in 2002–2003. The project was organised by a collaborative group of artists (Eriksson, Gunnars, Johnson, and Kindgren) that transformed the wards 109 and 110 at Ulleråker. Instead of focusing on a single artwork, they used their budget to improve the run-down facilities by changing furniture, fixing things that were broken, create direct access from the ward to the lawn outside, and similar actions. Today, there is little physical evidence left of the project since the ward is gone and what mainly remains is the documentation in a book published in 2006. This project was mainly interested in the institutional aspects of the history of the site. However, history can also be addressed by focusing on the former work and choreographies of the sites. This is the case in the project *Frenzie to Cure* (Botandes iver) which is a public art project by Maja Hammarén, who collaborated with the three other artists: Cecilia Germain, Ioana Cojocariu and Johanna Willenfelt. The first part of the project included a bus tour with three walking lectures and performative elements on sites in Gothenburg. The project has now moved on and will find a new form of expression in Uppsala and Ulleråker. In Gothenburg, the sites chosen were all in different ways related to how society treated or supervised problems such as poverty or mental distress, for example Lillhagen hospital. The participants involved, among others, people working on site. Together the participants helped recreate the choreography on site, the choreography of work or treatment. The performances deliberately functioned as a third time tool, "activating two layers of temporalities simultaneously", "walking through now-and-then-time in the same present" (Hammarén 2020). What remains of the project are the experiences of the artists, the participants and the people present on the site and what was related by the participants to other people.

6   Artistic Interventions

Rather than confirming time as something in which events take place, or that history inevitably repeats itself, many contemporary artists keep challenging official history, and investigates alternative plots. Something which can be done through the act of intervention. Such interventions are mainly done by problematizing the history of the institution or site, opening new, lost, or denied histories, challenging norms in relation to history by making them visible or by bringing new knowledge to the table. Not only does this bring new understanding, but it also adds something new and exciting that makes people want to explore and return to the site. Fred Wilson's exhibition *Mining the Museum* (1992–1993) at the Maryland Historical Society has been influential, inspiring numerous artistic interventions in museum institutions and historic sites. *Mining the Museum* helped expose both the history and norms of the institution and the visitor's relationship with the past. Wilson explains that he wanted to introduce histories that had been denied or lost. To invite the artist has become a way for the institution to open to self-examination and welcoming new perspectives on its collection and exhibition practices. Wilson's intention is to bring out the untold meanings hidden in collections and practices, not to replace the already existing ones but to let out the many different meanings an object carries (Wilson and Graham 2007, 214). The Museum of Medical History at Ulleråker has collaborated with contemporary artists on several occasions. For example, in the exhibition *Stoff. Konst på medicinhistoriska* (Medicinhistoriska museet 2017), with the artists Natasha Dahnberg (curator), Eva Högberg, Helena Laukkanen, Cecilia Levy, Moa Lönn (curator) and Katarina Sundkvist Zohari. The artworks were placed next to objects from the collection, establishing a dialogue with the objects on display. For example, in the exhibition catalogue, Cecilia Levy's artwork *Hjärnan* (The Brain) is placed next to an ECT-machine from the 1970s, designed for electroconvulsive therapy. The idea that materiality can carry memories and meanings is particularly relevant in places such as former mental institutions – where written or other records may be few and biased. These memories and meanings can be extracted when objects are placed in a carefully curated dialogue. Narratives are brought to life, involving different time layers, at least three: the points in time when the objects were made and used, when they were put together and the then when the two are experienced by the visitor. The fragile, sculptured brain made of paper and textile highlights the potentially destructive or healing power of the ECT-machine. Similarly, contemporary art could enter into a dialogue with patients' artwork.

7   The Tower

The Tower is a pre-study notebook (2018–2020) presented in a film by the artist Camille Norment. It takes its point of departure in material traces of the old water tower at Ulleråker. The tower contains a large empty water tank which becomes an inverted bell in the film and in an accompanying sound study. The water tank, no longer in use, has thus found a new application – no longer holding water but generating a sound that is speaking about past, present and future. Norment makes the bell's sound resonate through the different layers of time on site, with the intention to reveal both the visible and the mental state of the site (Norment 2020a). As Norment declares in her film, "When motions are deemed erratic, out of synch, they are cut from the mass. Time, place, perception, all become the same thing. They always were." (Norment 2020b, 1:34–1:50).

Norment's pre-study film does not tell a full story, there is no plot, there are only fragments, reverberations that have no beginning or end. Added to the bell sound there is the sound of water, once used for the treatment of patients, now the water in the ridge is threatened by the construction of new buildings. The film shows an old image of Ulleråker from the riverside. The text "Water was our fire – our pain and promise" is written over the image, suggesting to the many possible understandings of water (Norment 2020b, 9:04). There are also several images of old, tall trees in the film, many of which has to be cut down to make way for the new buildings and infrastructure. Norment writes over one of the images of trees: "Cut the trees so we can't breathe" (Norment 2020b, 7:08). In this way adding environmental critique to the study. By exploring her own experience of being accidentally locked in a car when first on her way to visiting the site, she is having us share her experience of involuntary confinement and panic, while also making us relate to earlier experiences of confinement on site. This connection to patient's experiences is enhanced in the film by images of keys made by former patients and exhibited in the museum. The keys, the experience of involuntary confinement, the sound, the site – all are given the opportunity to resonate within us, and in her film Norment talks about interconnectedness.

> Well, no it shouldn't suffice to be a historical tourist, you have to give something. Any history can be mediated by sound, they are both constantly in flux, always changing and subject to experience. (Norment 2020b, 12:00–13:43)

She also uses the concept of the *rhizome* to explain her relation to the site. Rhizome can be understood as "a metaphor of logic or conjunction that stresses nonlinear patterns of interconnection and feedback loops" (Barker 2004, 179). The post-structuralist concept was introduced by Gilles Deleuze and Félix Guattari in the book *A Thousand Plateaus: Capitalism and Schizophrenia* (1980). The rhizome is non-hierarchical, and history is understood as non-linear, without masterplan, beginning or end. In a rhizome all places can be connected, also different points in time. Norment uses sound, images and experience to help us connect to the rhizome and the past, present and future. This idea of connecting to the past resonates in the artwork *Parallel rooms*.

8   Parallel Rooms

Lies-Marie Hoffman's site-specific public artwork *Parallella rum* (Parallel rooms 2021, translation mine) is placed in the northeast part of Ulleråker, on a piece of land between the former fruit groves and the larger institution buildings seen on the edge of the ridge. You can see the sculpture from a distance, there are two portals, four benches, and the ground is covered with light gravel and cobbled stones. There is a choreography incorporated in the experience of

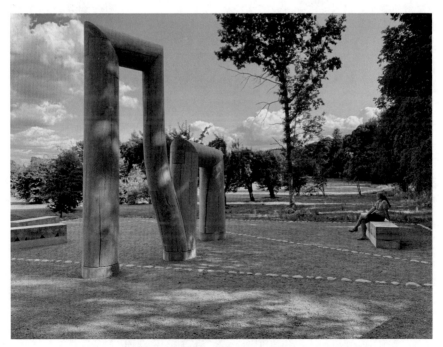

FIGURE 9.1   Lies-Marie Hoffman, The public artwork *Parallella rum* (Parallel rooms, 2021), Ulleråker, photo by Hedvig Mårdh

the work and you can move through, around and in the sculpture. The work is created from trees that were taken down to make room for new buildings, elm trees were used in the portals and larch was used to create the benches. Hoffman typically works with wood, and she is interested in sustainability.

Hoffman deliberately uses the artwork as a third-time tool and describes the work as having four dimensions, adding the dimension of time.

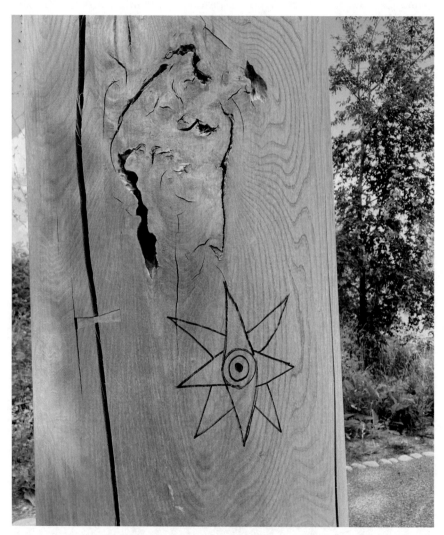

FIGURE 9.2   The Life of the artwork on site has begun, the star shape is an addition to the artwork made by an anonymous visitor. Lies-Marie Hoffman, *Parallella rum* (Parallel rooms, 2021), Ulleråker, photo by Hedvig Mårdh

The portal made of tree is an intersection between these dimensions, the small point through which time passes. The artwork challenges our fixation to linear events and offers us a different perspective, that different experiences of presence and time can exist simultaneously. (Uppsala kommun/Offentlig konst 2021, translation mine)

There are several time layers activated in this sculpture. The lifespan of the trees, the day they were cut down, the time of the site itself, the present – belonging to the people who visit, the duration of the choreography when you move in the sculpture, to mention a few. Moreover, the portals offer various framings of the surrounding area. Moving from one bench to the next you replace one frame for the next. Reflecting on the past you may focus on the fruit trees, planted, and cared for by patients or looking in the other direction you find the institutional building looming on the ridge. A huge nineteenth century building where patients have both suffered and found solvency, today it houses more than twenty artists. Passing through the portal, "the small point through which time passes" as Hoffman phrases it, there is a possibility of connecting the different layers, making them relevant in and for the present.

9   Conclusion

Art and artistic practices are increasingly used by, and integrated in, the management of complex heritage sites. The chapter specifically disscussed and analysed patients' art, urban exploration photography, exhibitions, public art and contemporary art in relation to the heritage of former mental healthcare institutions. Ricoeur's (1980), Fornäs' (2016) and Foucault's (1986) writings about time, narration and visual representations of the past have informed the analysis that show how artists use several different ways of approaching and narrating the past.

Photographers documenting abandoned and worn hospital buildings make use of the aesthetic potential of the sites, attracting visitors and creating an interest in preservation. Moreover, they often constitute the only documentation of the transformation of these sites. However, they also tend to confirm stereotypical representations of patients and psychiatry, and if we are looking to talk about the lives lived in these complex sites before the transformation, we need a variation of visual and spatial representations of the past and the people in it. Art, understood as third-time tools can help mediate between subjective and objective time creating cultural time (Fornäs 2016, 5215). The first approach to time according to Ricoeur, where art shows something of a datable, public, and measurable nature, is rare in the material analysed for this study.

The second approach, however, is more thematic and open for reflection. The curated dialogues between objects, patients' art from the past and contemporary art in the exhibition *Stoff* created a space for memories and meaning that usually have been lost because of the lack of written documents. Hoffman's work *Parallella rum* (2021) could also be seen to fit this second approach, although what she wishes to tell or teach us is less clear. Instead, by creating a "small point through which time passes", the work allows us to reflect on our connection to the people and actions that took up the space before us. Norment on the other hand consciously challenges the third approach, "the plot", the succession of events, making it clear that it does not suffice to be a historical tourist, you need to give something, thus wishing to create a reverberation that has nor beginning or end.

To conclude, art and professional artistic practices contribute to the mediation of the heritage of psychiatry. Artists create dialogues with the past, negotiate and occasionally challenge "objective history", "the plot" or how we relate to history. They do this by presenting alternatives to one-sided narratives about the past for the present, raising issues concerning power, norms, and stereotypes about mental health and the sites for treatment.

Acknowledgements

The research project *From Psychiatric Hospital to Condominium – Urban Development and Cultural Heritage* (2019–00589) was funded by Formas, a government research council for sustainable development.

References

Barker, Chris. "Rhizome." In *The SAGE Dictionary of Cultural Studies* 179. London: SAGE Publications Ltd, 2004. http://dx.doi.org.bibproxy.kau.se:2048/10.4135/978144 6221280.n209.

Bennett, Dawn, Anna Reid, and Peter Petocz. 2014. "Creative Workers' Views on Cultural Heritage and Sustainability." *Journal of Aesthetics & Culture* 6:1, 244–76.

Bourriaud, Nicolas. 2002. *Relational aesthetics*. Dijon: Presses du réel.

Cross, Simon. 2010. *Mediating Madness: Mental Distress and Cultural Representation*. Houndmills, Basingstoke, Hampshire: Palgrave Macmillan.

Franklin, Bridget. 2002. "Hospital – Heritage – Home: Reconstructing the Nineteenth Century Lunatic Asylum." *Housing, Theory and Society* 19:3–4, 170–184.

Fornäs, Johan. 2016. "The Mediatization of Third-Time Tools: Culturalizing and Histori-cizing Temporality." *International Journal of Communication* 10, 5213–5232.

Forsberg, Nils. 2022. "*Öppna* dörrar". *Dagens Nyheter.* 31 August.

Foucault, Michel. Translated by Miskowiec, Jay. 1986. "Of other spaces." *Diacritics* 16 (1): 22–27.

González-Sancho, Eva, and Per-Gunnar Eeg-Tverbakk. 2018. *Oslo Pilot (2015–17): A Project Investigating the Role of Art in and for Public Space – Laying the Groundwork for Oslo Biennial First Edition.* Milano: Mousse Publishing.

Hammarén, Maja. 2020. *Frenzie to Cure,* PDF sent to the author.

Hantelmann, Dorothea von. 2010. *How to Do Things With Art: What Performativity Means in Art.* Zürich: JRP Ringier.

Hartog, François. 2015. *Regimes of Historicity: Presentism and Experiences of Time,* Columbia University Press. ProQuest Ebook.

Hoffman, Ginger A.; and Jennifer L. Hansen. 2017. "Prozac Or Prosaic Diaries?: The Gendering of Psychiatric Disability in Depression Memoirs." *Philosophy, Psychiatry & Psychology* 24, no. 4: 285–298.

Jedvik, Hanna. 2018. "Vad händer med mentalsjukhuset Lillhagens kulturarv." *Kulturre-portaget i P1.* https://sverigesradio.se/sida/avsnitt/1211216?programid=767 (accessed December 10, 2019).

Jörnmark, Jan. 2007. *Övergivna platser.* Lund: Historiska Media.

Jörnmark, Jan. 2008. *Övergivna platser 2.* Lund: Historiska Media.

Magnusson, Ann and Uppsala kommun. 2017-11-27. *Konstprogram Ulleråker KUR-Konst Ulleråker, Tema: Farvatten – droppa, forsa, stänk.* https://www.uppsala.se /kommun-och-politik/publikationer/konstprogram-ulleraker-kur/.

Medicinhistoriska museet. 2017. *Stoff. Konst på medicinhistoriska.*

Metzger, Jonathan. 2011. "Strange Spaces: A Rationale for Bringing Art and Artists into the Planning Process." *Planning Theory* 10:3, 213–238.

Moon, Graham, Robin Kearns, and Alun Joseph. 2015. *The Afterlives of the Psychiatric Asylum: Recycling Concepts, Sites and Memories.* Farnham, Surrey: Ashgate.

Övergivna platser. https://www.facebook.com/groups/11027840069/ (accessed July 6, 2021).

Ricoeur, Paul. 1980. "Narrative Time". *Critical Inquiry* 7:1, Autumn. 169–190.

SVT, Anders Nordqvist. 2017. „Kuslig konst på Beckomberga ska rivas". https://www.svt.se/nyheter/lokalt/stockholm/kuslig-konst-pa-beckomberga-ska-rivas. (accessed February 20, 2017).

Tate. Undated. Art term: Relational Aesthetics. https://www.tate.org.uk/art/art-terms /r/relational-aesthetics. (accessed September 20, 2020).

Uppsala kommun. 2015. Planprogram för Ulleråker. Samrådshandling, samrådstid 15 juni till 4 september. Plan och byggnadsnämnden, juni 2015. Dnr: PBN 2012-20250.

(accessed September 1, 2020). https://www.uppsala.se/contentassets/85c419fb5fdd4e9491e6a349b56e068d/ulleraker_handling_webb.pdf

Uppsala kommun/Offentlig konst. April 2021. Instagram *offentligkonstuppsalakommun*. (accessed July 6, 2021).

Wilson, A. Fred, and A. Mark Graham. 2007. "An Interview with Artist Fred Wilson." *The Journal of Museum Education* 32(3):211–219.

CHAPTER 10

Re-Assembling the Social in So Called "Mental Illness"? Reflections on the Uses of Material Culture in the Historiography of Psychiatry and in Mad Studies

Elena Demke

Abstract

While the significance of things in the "making of patients" and the ways in which patients appropriated their role in the material surroundings of psychiatric care have attracted increasing interested by cultural historians, the story of materiality in experiences of madness and recovery outside its psychiatric definition has remained largely untold.

My chapter will talk about a project that constitutes a first attempt to fill this gap. Funded by the German ministry of research and education, and relying on ethical and epistemological considerations of survivor research and Mad Studies, a "virtual museum of madness and recovery/discovery" is being created. Based on "object-elicited interviews", psychiatric survivors in Germany tell their stories of madness and recovery, focusing on things that acquired special meanings during experiences of crises and the struggles to come to terms with them. The things that come into focus include objects facilitating protection and helpful bonds such as dolls or personal talismans, stories about special meanings attached to food and clothing during crises up to visions or the power of ordering and re-ordering things in one's daily life. Rituals that enable persons to find their personal path through extreme distress receive special attention in these narratives. They can be understood outside pathologizing categories when research sticks to tracing the "agency of the objects" in interrelation with the agency of the person using them. While these things and their usages speak about attempts to tackle unusual, and often scary or traumatic situations, the materiality of psychiatry focuses on "fixing the person". Thus, the focus on materiality here helps to juxtapose the medical and the social model of disability as applied to mental crises.

My chapter will not only discuss the findings from 20 interviews with psychiatric survivors but also discuss the methodology of the research: How is survivor-control facilitated? How does it affect the interviewing and the conceptualizing and planning of a virtual museum? When the classical pitfalls in terms of epistemological

© KONINKLIJKE BRILL BV, LEIDEN, 2025 | DOI:10.1163/9789004519848_012

injustice are being addressed – to what extend can knowledge production and the public representation of marginalized experiences ever be just?

Keywords

Mad Studies – *MAD Museum anderer Dinge* – materiality – object-elicited interviews – survivor control

While the significance of things in the 'making of patients' and the ways in which patients appropriated their roles within the material assemblages of psychiatry have attracted growing interest by historians of psychiatry (e.g. Majerus and Ankele 2020; Coleborne 2014), materiality in experiences of mental crises, madness and recovery outside their psychiatric definitions did not attract similar interest. On the one hand, this is surprising. Considering the intellectual indebtedness of the material turn in the humanities to traditions of thought which question dichotomies such as modern versus non-modern, material versus immaterial, rational versus irrational,[1] and the connectedness of some of its proponents with postcolonial theorizing, it seems an obvious step from here to try and look at madness as an experience not to be equaled with patienthood or mental illness. On the other hand, this is not surprising at all. Although diagnoses have been historicized and their social and political implications been de-constructed (e.g. Bernet 2013; Herrn 2022; Schmiedebach 2016), the hegemonic medical narrative that equals madness and illness has persisted. In the last consequences and in contradiction to their own deconstructivist claims, historians have continued to follow it, often equaling the "history of psychiatry" with the "history of madness".

As the trajectories of various anti-discrimination movements show, the overcoming of hegemonic narratives is not a matter of turns and twists but one of continual work. Conceptualizing the materiality of madness and recovery[2] as distinct from the material cultures of psychiatry can be a step on this path. This also implies to think in terms of a "material heritage of madness"[3] as distinct from that of psychiatry.

---

1   This applies to some of the most prominent authors of the "material turn" such as Latour, Miller, Appadurai et al.
2   The term is here understood as originally developed by the survivor movement (see Penney, and Prescott 2016).
3   Hence the title of the 2019 conference paper this chapter is based on: "Same objects – no common language. Why we should distinguish between material cultures of madness and material cultures of psychiatry."

Of course, 'heritage' depends on cultures they 'preserve' – and co-constitute – and talking of madness as being cultural, in an era in which the abundance of research relating to experiences qualified as "mad" aims at tackling brain dysfunctions is challenging. Mad Studies which originated from the movement of (ex-)users and survivors of psychiatry has taken up this challenge most decidedly.

This chapter addresses the interface of material culture studies and Mad Studies. To do so, I will first discuss the ways in which materiality has been addressed so far by Mad Studies and related approaches by scholars who explicate their perspectives as rooted in experiences of madness and psychiatric reactions to it, and contrast this with research on the material cultures of psychiatry without such explicit positionality. In a second step, I will discuss methodological insights and first findings from a project that has tried to take the use of material culture approaches in Mad Studies a step further, relying on object-focused interviewing and survivor-control in studying the meanings of things in experiences of crisis, madness and psychiatric reactions to them and in eventually creating a digital museum which went online in October 2022 under the title of MAD_Museum Anderer Dinge.[4] Throughout, I will discuss the effects the various ways to focus on materiality have on the emerging narratives.

1   Materiality in Mad Studies vs. in the Historiography of Psychiatry

Mad Studies' academic and activist cradle was in Toronto/Canada (Lefrançois et al. 2013; Church and Reville 2012), however, boundaries with (ex-)user/ survivor research (Sweeney et al. 2009) and with research activities by psychiatric survivors and allies explicating their perspectivity but using none of these terms are fluid. These strands of research taken together, the number of scholars relying on mad experience as an explicit aspect of their heuristics appears as relatively small – for obvious reasons with respect to the stigma associated.

Given this marginal situation and the scarcity of funding, the work on material histories by mad-identified scholars is considerable: Activism and scholarship of one of the founding authors of Mad Studies, historian Geoffrey Reaume, have been dedicated to questions of materiality right from the beginning, focusing, among others, on former hospital walls not only as materialization of patients' labour and hence as commemorative sites but also as spaces of contemporary interventions. Thus, during guided tours, former

---

4   Museummandererdinge.de (accessed January 31, 2023).

patients disclosed their identity and shared their knowledge on masonry, and institutional regimes concerning patient labour, effectively disrupting clichés of (non-)expertise.[5] The Mad Studies stream offered at the School of Disability Studies at Ryerson University, Toronto, includes courses on "Mad People's history" and "History of Madness" as well as the methodology of working with material sources (Landry and Church, 2016). Its director, Kathryn Church, not only curated an exhibition which integrated Mad and Disability History (Church et al. 2018) but also encouraged scholarship transcending disciplinary boundaries of art versus social science (Reid et al. 2019). The 2004 Master thesis by Jijian Voronka, who by now is one of the very few university professors rooted in Mad Studies, dealt with the material agency as well as the discursive significance of (former) mental hospital buildings in Ontario, Canada (Voronka 2004). Furthermore, the very first Master's degree in Mad Studies[6] which was recently launched at the Queen's University of Edinburgh, has been built upon courses on "Mad People's History and Identity". In environments less favourable to mad perspectives entering the academia, grass-root activism has addressed the significance of material sites, nonetheless. Thus, in Germany, the Irrenoffensive e.v. ('lunatics' offensive'), together with the Bund der Psychiatrie-Erfahrenen, BPE e.v. ('Federation of Survivors of Psychiatry') campaigned to set up a "Museum der wahnsinnigen Schönheit" ('museum of mad beauty') in Berlin's Tiergartenstraße, at the site of the organizing of the patient-killings under Nazi rule, years before a state and citizen initiative eventually launched a memorial site (Hinz-Wessels 2015; Demke 2024). Apparently, interest in material histories and scholarship as well as activism redressing stigma and the exclusion of mad perspectives have been closely intertwined.

It can be argued, that these activities – together with the sharing of testimonials, traditions of survivor-controlled forms of peer support and the trajectories of decades of collective human rights activism – give shape to an emerging cultural memory (Assmann, 2011) of the mad movement. The material focus of this memory seemingly deals with the 'same' things which historians consider elements of the 'material culture of psychiatry'. However, since mad cultural memory constitutes a different context, the significance of these things radically differs, too. Therefore assuming a 'material culture of madness' as distinct from that of psychiatry may be an useful clarification.

---

5   http://activehistory.ca/papers/historypaper-10/#WALLTOURS (accessed March 20 2021).
6   See https://www.qmu.ac.uk/news-and-events/news/2020/20201130-qmu-launches-the-world-s-first-master-s-in-mad-studies/ (accessed July 24 2023).

The following example of a project that re-assembled (Latour 2007) the social world of mad biographies, and the discussion of its reception by scholarship focusing the material culture of psychiatry may further illuminate the significance of this difference. In 1998, activist and social scientist Darby Penney, together with psychiatrist and ally Peter Stastny, learned about 427 suitcases that had been found at the attic of the Willard mental hospital, Upstate New York, filled with personal possessions of former inmates most of whom had spent decades of their lives and eventually died at Willard (Penny and Stastny 2009). The suitcases were the material reminders of their lives before patienthood. Lacking funding for a systematic research on all suitcases and their owners, Penney and Stastny selected 25 for further exploration following an intuitive heuristic, choosing those "that called out to us in a loud and clear manner" (*ibid.*, 17), including one suitcase that stood out for the scarcity of its content. Items of originally practical use – cutlery, pottery, clothing – had been preserved along with commemorabilia such as postcards, letters and photos. Matching the patient files of former owners with the contents of the suitcases, Penny and Stastny re-assembled meaningful biographies, as in the example of a man whose patient file mentioned the death of his wife and baby, and who had stored in his suitcase a dried brides' bouquet and decorated dress. Adding up of hardships such as orphanage, migration, poverty or early bereavement were characteristic of all the biographies researched. Among them, there was Margaret D., a specialist nurse who spent 32 years as an inpatient at Willard and whose trunk had "by far, the largest accumulation of personal possessions among the suitcase owners" (*ibid.*, 84). Letters, postcards, diplomas, a driving licence and many more objects allowed Penney and Stastny to trace the hardships (early death of both parents, death of her fiancé) and personal strengths which characterized Margaret's life (a girl growing up in an orphan house in Scotland around 1900 securing her education against the odds, migrating to the US, and living an independent life as a single working woman) as well as the "escalating cumulation of stress" preceding her involuntary admission to Willard which led to rapid deterioration. Thus, together with information from files, the things from the suitcases take on the meanings of 'symptoms' of alternative 'diagnoses', resonant with what can be considered the core formula of numerous narratives of ex-patients/survivors: "broken hearts, not broken brains".[7]

While the resulting book does not come along as an academic piece of work – no referencing, no explicit use of theory – the procedure of research

---

7   This formula was termed by Dolly Sen, e.g. in Demke/Olostiak-Brahms 2019, 82, see also: https://wellcomecollection.org/series/XmifPBIAAB8Ae-b4 (accessed March 15 2021).

evokes urban ethnology in the vein of, for example, Daniel Miller (Miller 2011): Things are understood as the stuff subjectivities were made from, subjectivities which psychiatric diagnostics and treatment did not grasp and appreciate. A sharp contrast between despair made tangible through material traces of lost hopes and the inhumane since unempathic psychiatric intervention is the core plot of the resulting narrative. The authors do not shy away from framing their conclusion as a statement addressing a fundamental issue of mental health care: "If someone had taken the time and the effort to piece together these people's stories during their lifetimes, [this] ... might have led to a successful resumption of the lives they led before being institutionalized." (Penney and Stastny 2009, 20).

The reception of this work by historians who focus on the material culture of psychiatry underlines the differences between activist and academic scholarship. While it has been called "stunning" (Coleborne 2017, 35) or "impressive [and] stimulating" (Majerus and Ankele 2020, 14), the difference in approach and conclusions and its striving for re-assembling the social in 'mental illness' and thereby questioning the very concept of medicalizing psychological distress is not taken up and nor is it addressed in citing this work in the sense of embarking on a discourse.

A recent collection of historiographical chapters and art work on "material cultures of psychiatry" (Majerus and Ankele 2020) includes pencil contour drawing of items from the Willard suitcases. Inspired by the adaption of the suitcase project by a photographer, this art work inverts the interest in biographies of the former: It combines items from suitcases of various owners with drawings of a straightjacket, a strap for fixation, bathtubs and other institutional objects and it uses Margaret's patient file number[8] as a title without making reference to the person. Such an "autonomous iconography of the object" (Barthes 1980, 23) frustrates interest in information. This can generate a productive tension, in particular, when dealing with overly familiar contexts and when wishing to disrupt all-to-easy-made associations. However, with respect to psychiatric patients, such as patient 25682 whose identity as Margaret D. had been restored by Darbey and Penney (2009), the situation is inverted: Here, the very absence of context is the familiar and the stereotype, and reconstructing the biography amounts to the productive disruption by activist researchers. Such a restoring of context is political since it refers to the inhumanity of a treatment ignoring social hardships and their effects on biographies.

---

8   See also: https://www.post-gazette.com/news/health/2010/09/01/Life-of-Margaret-D-25682 /stories/201009010171 (accessed March 25 2021).

Thus, this de-contextualization of the Willard suitcase project in the context of a publication on "material cultures of psychiatry" appears less as an effect of art work versus historiography than as one of the different heuristic framings constituted by thinking in terms of a 'material culture of madness' versus one of psychiatry.

Studies in the material culture of psychiatry are interested in the agency of people in patient roles but tend not ask what is at stake in psychiatry. The uses of material objects in the works by conventional historians of psychiatry and proponents of Mad Studies lead to very different narratives: While the former understand things as signs of unspecific human agency, they are read as signs of oppression and resistance by the latter. This implies narratives which 'discover' patients as humans on the one hand in contrast to those which strive to honour them as victims and resisters on the other. Accordingly, the material assemblages studied become a stage on which different types of performances are made visible.

Ways of addressing materiality	Studies in material cultures of psychiatry	Mad Studies and related activist scholarship
Things are traces of	unspecified human agency	oppression and resistance
Patients are	discovered as humans	commemorated and honoured as victims and resisters
Material assemblages of psychiatry are	sites of negotiation, appropriation	sites of oppression and exploitation

2   Researching the Meanings of Things in Experiences of Distress, Madness and Psychiatric Reaction to Them

In conclusion, by focusing materiality, Mad Studies have addressed aspects of the interaction of society, psychiatry and the mad and questioned the construct of mental illness by providing social context. However, so far they have made little use of theories related to the 'material turn' in the humanities and have not dealt with the meaning of things in experiences of madness. History of psychiatry, in contrast, uses the respective theories, is interested in how patients made sense of their environments, but not in how they made sense of madness.

The second half of this chapter introduces a project addressing this gap, drawing on survivor-led research in the vein of Mad Studies as well as insights of the Actor-Network theory to explore the meanings of things in experiences of crisis, madness and psychiatric reactions to them.

For so doing, it uses theoretical framings provided by the material turn as well as by Mad Studies. It holds that what is at stake in psychiatry is the contested capacity of the mad in meaning-making and that therefore mad people's agency in this particular respect, is of central significance.

It began from personal experience and narratives shared by peers on stealing things from psychiatric institutions: stealing one's patient file and using it for a book about one's journey through madness and the effects of various types of psychiatries on it (Kempker 2000), stealing a glass which had served for delivering medication and using it for beverages (Transcript O), stealing a towel with a year of personal significance – denied by psychiatric interpretation – printed on it (Transcript U), stealing institutional clothing and going to a carnival as a 'madman' soon after (Transcript M). Such acts of self-assertion and subversion are not primarily about negotiating one's position in a psychiatric institution but they target issues of meaning-making and strive to subvert the power relations controlling it. Since supposedly deficient ways of handling meaning are at the core of the allocation of diagnoses of 'severe mental illness', mad people's agency in terms of meaning-making appears particularly significant, beyond that of navigating institutional constraints.

Based on these observations, a broader research question emerged: how do people deal with meanings of things in situations of crisis and adversary[9]? This broadened question was applied to case studies from different times and cultures in an interdisciplinary joined research project.[10] The project focusing on distress, madness and psychiatric reactions to it, was conducted as one of these case studies, based on interviews with and autoethnographic writings by (ex-)users and survivors of psychiatry in Germany. The second part of this chapter discusses some of its methodological and theoretical considerations which are understood as part of the work that is needed to divert from the hegemonic narrative of distress and madness as 'mental illness'. Put in a nutshell, these assumptions are:

a. Since tellability shapes what can be known and tellability depends on social resonance, a peer-setting changes the epistemology.

b. The agency of things, if allowed to unfold, may productively disrupt role expectations in research.

---

9   Funded by the German ministry of research and education (BMBF).

10   https://www.sisi.uni-bonn.de/projekt (accessed March 20 2021).

c.   'Black boxed' meanings which tend to be taken for granted, have to be de_scribed in order to transcend the medical gaze on the materiality of psychiatry.

3   Collaboration and (Ex-)User Control: Sharing Risks and Power

The effect of shared backgrounds on telling stories of stigmatized experience can hardly be overestimated. Thus, a study about deaf women's exposure to violence found that the incidence reported nearly tripled (Schröttle 2015), when interviews were conducted by peers. Obviously, a peer setting shifts the limits of tellability. In the context of a large-scale, collaborative project on social suffering in contemporary society, based on interviews conducted in the outskirts of Paris, Pierre Bourdieu analysed this phenomenon as a reducing or even removing of the threats of objectivation since interviewee and inter-viewer share, "by the same token, the risks of that exposure" (Bourdieu 1999, 611). While Bourdieu referred to social proximity in general, this effect seems to be even more significant when stigma is at stake. Since medical discourse con-siders the impossibility of interpersonal understanding as a defining feature of madness, an understanding based on shared mad experience implies a radi-cal departure from that dooming. Survivor Research and Mad Studies, while also warning of the risks of co-optation and reductionism involved (Voronka 2019), have long recognized the vital role of sharing stories. 'Safe spaces' that rely on the willingness to divert from common views on the defective mind of mad people allow for striving for an understanding "on our own terms" (e.g. Wallcraft et al. 2003). While this has always been relevant to interpersonal encounters in independent peer-support, User/Survivor research and Mad Studies have built upon these dynamics in order to produce a new knowledge on mental distress, challenging the medical paradigm.

Applied to researching material culture, the strife to gain an understanding 'on our own terms' implies that terminologies are open to be negotiated, and so are interpretations, since those who define meaning have the power (Hodder 2013). This is not just an ethical demand but an epistemological tool. Thus, the call for interviews left it open to the interviewee to define what constitutes 'a thing'. As a result, a fluid boundary between the material and the immaterial was assumed, since different attitudes to these boundaries became obvious. Thus, an interviewee informed me that it seemed utterly unsuitable to her, to speak of a 'thing' with respect to the doll which she chose as the focus of her interview (Transcript E), whereas to another interviewee a vision constituted a 'thing' in the sense of the research question (Transcript E). These assumptions divert from conventional Western ontologies, in a way which fits, not the talking of 'sick minds', but epistemological claims of the material turn. Without following these diversions it would be impossible to grasp and appreciate how things become helpful or detrimental in trying to establish agency in situations of extreme distress.

4   From 'Elicitation' to Encounter: Methodological Framing of
        Interviews Focusing Material Cultures of Madness

In this project, a range of things were put forward by interviewees and their meaningful handling in relation to experiences of distress and madness has been the focus of a shared exploration by the interviewee and the interviewer. Interviews dealt with their materiality, origin, acquisition, practices of handling and storing them.

The methodology was inspired by the method of 'object-elicitation' which in turn draws on 'photo-elicited research' (e.g. Harper 2002). Although overlapping with the material turn, object elicitation does not necessarily focus on material culture and the meanings and handlings of objects, but may be confined to using objects for generating narratives. In this sense, object-elicitation has been explicitly used in researching the way patients suffering from terminal cancer deal with anticipated loss (Willig 2016), and similarly, so called 'identity-boxes' have been used to explore the construction of identity under conditions of chronical illness (fibromyalgia) (Brown 2019). However, objects not only elicit narratives but if present in the research setting, their agency unfolds in the interaction, too. In a research context that tries to question power relations, this is especially valuable. While a shared identity as (ex-) users/survivors of psychiatry may remove the 'threats of objectivation' in the above sense, the distribution of roles in an interview is another power-loaden issue. However, things can come into play to the effect of re-negotiating power relations and thereby enhance the scope of understanding.

One instance was particularly instructive in this respect (Transcript F). On the first contact, by telephone, an interviewee had given me the impression that she[11] did not embrace the focus on the meanings of objects. I put an emphasis on this aspect in the preliminary talk, assuming that an interview merely focusing on a biographical narrative would not serve the research

---

11   In this text, the female pronoun is used throughout in order to stick with the standards of anonymity agreed upon for the MAD_Museum Anderer Dinge. There, the gender of narratives can be chosen by visitors, but the actual gender of interviewees remains anonymous.

question. When I met the interviewee at his home, she had prepared a set of 12 small things – photos, figures, certificates – sitting on a desk, each accompanied by a decoratively numbered button. She explained that these things stood for important steps in her life and went on telling the interviewer about her biography, characterized by early orphanhood, material hardship and lacking support for her education, mental crises leading to periods as a psychiatric inpatient and long times of dullying medication, followed by her struggle to gain control of her life and commitment in the survivor movement. The figures symbolizing stages of this biography – such as a duck for awkward teenage times, a leaflet for becoming vegan, an empty tablet box for getting off neuroleptics – had been chosen for the purpose of the interview but held no particular significance for her beyond that.

Looking for things that had been meaningful in crises, had granted agency or materialized special memories, these objects did not seem to fit the research question. Futile questions in the early stage of the interview document my hesitation to fully engage with the interviewee and to adapt my research outlook to what she had to tell (Transcript F). However, in the course of the encounter which entailed more than one meeting, the significance of this narrative became increasingly clear. The interviewee had in her home also things which she had acquired in times of distress. These were rather unusual and, without the context of her biographical narrative, may have offered themselves easily to pathologizing interpretation. However, through materializing stages of her biographical narrative, the interviewee had provided an option to be understood on her own terms. Only against her biographical account, the meaning of those special things became feasible.

Only a few more findings from this project can be addressed in this chapter. They were selected for the purpose of underlining the usefulness of the material turn for questioning the medical gaze.

5   Mad Agency in the Material Environment of the Institution

Human agency requires command over things. Narratives of experiencing madness and patienthood poignantly point towards this simple and yet vital insight. In her memoirs on her experience with psychoses and psychiatric reaction towards them, Norwegian author and psychologist Arnhild Lauveng, born 1974, describes being in an isolation room, in Norway in the 1990s. Deprived of any means that she might possibly have used to hurt herself, she took to tearing off the wall paper with her teeth (Lauveng 2010, 95). To medical staff, this appeared as yet another symptom of her 'schizophrenia' while in her book, she explains she had been an outraged and angry teenager wanting to do *some-thing*. Being in an empty room with her hands tied, tearing of wallpaper with her teeth was one of the few remaining options. Thus, once the pathological gaze is dropped, mad actions appear to make sense. German sculptor, activist and survivor of forced sterilization under Nazism, Dorothea Buck (1917–2019) described in her memoirs how, being a young woman fearing sexual assault in a psychiatric hospital in the 1930s, she defecated into her bed on purpose – hoping the smell might deter intruders (Buck-Zerchin 2016, 64).

While E. Goffman famously argued that any actions by patients, also those that are considered 'normal' in daily life, are considered symptoms of mental illness due to effects of the 'total institution' (Goffman 1990, 1961), first person accounts on the handling of things under involuntary hospitalization show that the inversion applies, too: supposedly 'abnormal' acting appears as logical under institutional constraints limiting possibilities for handling emotional distress. While these examples concern questions of negotiating the psychiatric space, a material culture perspective allows us also to move further towards overcoming the medical gaze.

6   De_Scribing Objects of Psychiatry: the Example of Neuroleptics

The social agency of one of the core objects of psychiatry since the 2nd half of the 20th century – neuroleptics – may serve as an example. For the purpose of this chapter, the focus will be on actions involving the rejection of neuroleptics.

In the context of studying the ways in which, upon their introduction in the 1950s, neuroleptics changed routines, uses of space, rhythms and interactions, historian Majerus interpreted instances of their rejection by patients as expressing resistance to a perceived "negative power of doctors" (Benoit Majerus 2016, 61) or "opposition to hospitalization" (*ibid.*, 58). This interpretation rests on the meaning inscribed to these pills and injections by psychiatry. If the medical gaze is to be overcome, it needs to be historicized, or, in the terminology of the ANT, de_scribed.

At this point a rather superficial reference to the ANT has to suffice to make the point concerning its heuristic power (see Belliger et al. 2006). In this perspective, neuroleptics became tested and enrolled in an action programme involving the material agent 'neuroleptic drugs' with human actors such as producers, medical stuff, families and people in the roles of patients to the end of 'treating mental illness'. Majerus' observation from the times of their introduction, according to which a considerable number of patients were opposed to taking them, together with the fact that involuntary neuroleptic medication has been relentlessly controversial since (e.g. Lehmann 2019, 2010; Balz 2010) thus can be framed as an instability of patients' mobilization in this action programme. Accordingly, the meaning of 'medication' which appears as 'black boxed' for mobilized actors, is not taken for granted by people in patient roles that resist them.

Survivor and peer worker Gwen Schulz wrote about her attitudes to, handling of and reflection on neuroleptics (e.g. Schulz 2008). Since her first hospitalization as a teenager she had resented the neuroleptics she was given, feeling deprived of her dignity by their numbing effects, leading to uncontrolled salivation, hampered ability to walk, and dullness. In the course of one of her inpatient stays later on, injections were replaced by tablets, giving her the opportunity to secretly spit them out. Unwittingly, through this action, she 'enrolled' neuroleptics in a different testing. Months after her secretive stopping of taking them, doctors officially announced the reduction of her medication. From then on, staff commented that she deteriorated due to the supposed process of tempering off. Knowing that there was no tempering off, she began to wonder about the significance of medication for doctors and nurses. She understood it as a kind of placebo effect for medical staff. In the terminology of the ANT, she de_scribed the medical meaning of neuroleptics.

But what did the rejection of neuroleptics mean to her? G. Schulz talks about diverting from the idea of fighting symptoms and instead including them in her concept of self. This way, harrowing experiences such as hearing voices of contemptuous and threatening content did not cease, but became more manageable, sparing her a continuation of repeated hospitalisation.

Other narrations of rejecting neuroleptics point towards a similar interpretation. Thus rituals of throwing away tablets (Transcripts Q, U) became a kind of rites des passage towards embracing one's mad self, and accepting suffering. Seen this way, 'rejecting psychiatry' appears as an inevitable side effect, but not as the fundamental significance of these actions.

7   Mad Agency: a Doll that Blurs the Boundary between the Material and Immaterial, an Axe that May as Well Be a Hammer, a Sandwich that Enshrines Mad Competence and Solidarity

Rejecting things that are deemed unsuitable by the individual user – such as neuroleptics in the above example – are one side of the coin in accepting suffering and striving for personal ways to cope, the other side is finding personal things enhancing one's agency. Many of such usages of things under extreme mental distress have been pathologized. Thus, psychologist Habermas speaks of an immature, regressive way of using objects and a loss of reality when a material object becomes more important to the user than interhuman relationships (Habermas 1999).

Out of 20 interviews from this project,[12] three dealt with dolls as a central topic. At least two of them stereotypically seem to fulfil Habermas' criteria, being permanent companions to their adult owners, and being addressed and talked about in ways similar to inter-human dyads. Among them there is a doll called Margot, owned by the writer Nicoleta Craita Ten'O[13] who gave up using spoken language when she was 13 years old, together with her decision "to stay a child forever" (Transcript H). The first interview with her, I conducted at her home, using written language. On a second occasion, our communication was confined to gestures and body language. Relying on these means of communication, our exchange was vivid. After her dog had accidentally hurt me, the interviewee caressed my superficially wounded hand, hugged me and apologized using an attentive, caring body language.

Attributions of 'immaturity' and 'loss of reality' appear out of place in the face of such attentiveness, caring manner and the ability to anticipate questions of the interviewer. Instead, the challenge Nicoleta faces, is to be taken seriously. Her wish no to grow up and to reject a brutal adult world may be well-grounded, and doll Margot be part of putting it into practice.

While her muteness and permanent carrying of Margot seems to fit the clichés of the diagnoses attributed to her, her caring manner, empathizing with my needs and her reflections that seemed to anticipate my question spoke a different language.

Thus she pointed out that there had been experiences of violence and transgression motivating her decision "not to grow up" but added that she did not wish to elaborate on this. After having spent some time with Nicoleta, it occurred to me that performing the resolution "not to become an adult" is a permanent challenge, to which always carrying the doll Margot may be an answer. And who finds himself in a position to call the decision to dismiss a brutal adult world "a loss of reality"?

This applies in particular to those objects which in public perception are easily associated with the stereotype of the dangerous, aggressive mad person. One interviewee talked about carrying an axe with herself for months (Transcript L): an older, but well functioning axe which she had bought at a flea market, impressed by its traditional appearance. She had enjoyed using it for wood work, but at a time of distress, she began to carry it permanently, fixed to her belt, and hidden underneath a rug which she wore in place of a coat. Now, the axe took on a new meaning, symbolizing protection against bad influence. A neighbour became aware of the axe and the dangers carrying it entailed and addressed the issue, asking whether another tool might serve the same purpose. Together they found a small glaziers hammer that replaced the axe. The

12   Of March 2021.
13   Most recent publication at the time of the interview: Craita Ten'o 2018.

fact that the greater force of the axe as a potential weapon did not matter to the owner refers to the meaning it held for her, and which remarkably differs from the association with danger and aggression commonly ascribed to such an instrument.

Understanding mad meanings of things may also create agency in terms of being able to support others. One interviewee had known fears of being poisoned during her times of distress (Transcript K). Later on, she trained to work in peer support.[14] In this context, she worked at a ward where medical staff was worried about a woman who kept refusing to eat. The interviewee asked for permission to try to help in her way. Assuming that the woman in question was hungry but deterred from eating by fears similar to those which she had experienced, she knelt down on the floor and took steps to share a meal. She prepared a sandwich and suggested to take bites in turns: And indeed, it worked, and the woman at risk began to eat.

Insight into the material culture of madness may enhance understanding – this may also hold true for historians who wish to overcome the medical gaze. Mad actions can be understood beyond pathologizing categories when the research sticks to tracing the 'agency of the objects' in interrelation with the agency of the person using them. The emerging narratives no longer focus on persons that need fixing but on tackling unusual, and often scary or traumatic situations. Used this way, the focus on materiality can contribute to re-assembling the much neglected social in so called mental illness.

References

Ankele, Monika, and Benoît Majerus, eds. 2020. *Material Cultures of Psychiatry*. Bielefeld: Transcript.

Assmann, Aleida. 2011. *Cultural Memory and Western Civilization: Functions, Media, Archives*. New York: Cambridge University Press.

Balz, Viola. 2010. *Zwischen Wirkung Und Erfahrung: Eine Geschichte Der Psychopharmaka: Neuroleptika in Der Bundesrepublik Deutschland, 1950–1980*. Bielefeld: Transcript.

Barthes, Roland. 2000. *A Barthes Reader*. Vintage.

Belliger, Andréa, and David J. Krieger, eds. 2006. *ANThology: Ein Einführendes Handbuch zur Akteur-Netzwerk-Theorie*. Bielefeld: Transcript.

Bernet, Brigitta. 2013. *Schizophrenie: Entstehung und Entwicklung eines psychiatrischen Krankheitsbilds um 1900*. Zürich: Chronos.

Bourdieu, Pierre, and Alain Accardo, eds. 1999. *The Weight of the World: Social Suffering in Contemporary Society*. Stanford: Stanford University Press.

---

14   See https://ex-in.de/ (accessed March 22, 2021).

Brown, Nicole. 2019. "Identity Boxes: Using Materials and Metaphors to Elicit Experiences." *International Journal of Social Research Methodology* 22 (5): 487–501.

Buck-Zerchin, Dorothea S. 2016. *Auf der Spur des Morgensterns: Psychose als Selbstfindung*. Neumünster: Paranus. (6th edition).

Church, Kathryn, Melanie Panitch, Catherine Frazee, and Phaedra Livingstone. 2018. "'Out from Under': A Brief History of Everything." In *Untold Stories: A Canadian Disability History Reader*, edited by Nancy Hansen, Roy Hanes, and Diane Driedger, 8–25. Toronto: Canadian Scholars Press.

Coleborne, Catharine, and Dolly MacKinnon, eds. 2017. *Exhibiting Madness in Museums: Remembering Psychiatry through Collections and Display*. London: Routledge.

Craita Ten'o, Nicoleta. 2018. *Die Naht des Silberschuhs: ein Jugendroman*. Vechta-Langförden: Geest-Verlag.

Demke, Elena and Mirko Olostiak-Brahms. 2019. *Psychose als Selbstfindung. Bald 100 Stimmen zu Dorothea Bucks 100. Geburtstag*. Bochum: bpe.

Demke, Elena. 2024. Contested Memorialization: Filling the 'Empty Space' of the T4 Murders. In Sites of Conscience. Place, Memory and the Project o Deinstitutionalization, edited by Elisabeth Punzi and Linda Steele, 46-63. Vancouver: UBC Press.D

Goffman, Erving. 1990. *Asylums: Essays on the Social Situation of Mental Patients and Other Inmates*. New York: Doubleday.

Habermas, Tilmann. 2012. *Geliebte Objekte: Symbole und Instrumente der Identitätsbildung*. Frankfurt am Main: Suhrkamp. (2nd edition).

Harper, Douglas. 2002. "Talking about Pictures: A Case for Photo Elicitation." *Visual Studies* 17 (1): 13–26.

Herrn, R. 2022. "Aushandlungen einer reichseinheitlichen psychiatrischen Klassifikation oder wie aus dem Berliner Schlüssel der Würzburger Schlüssel wurde." *Medizinhistorisches Journal* 57 (1): 36–73.

Hinz-Wessels, Annette. 2015. *Tiergartenstrasse 4: Schaltzentrale der nationalsozialistischen "Euthanasie"-Morde*. Berlin: Links.

Hodder, Ian, ed. 2013. *The Meanings of Things*. London: Routledge.

Kempker, Kerstin. 2000. *Mitgift: Notizen vom Verschwinden*. Berlin: Antipsychiatrieverlag.

Latour, Bruno. 2007. *Reassembling the Social: An Introduction to Actor-Network-Theory*. Oxford: Oxford University Press.

Landry, Danielle, and Kathryn Church. 2016. "Teaching (like) Crazy in a Mad Positive School: Exploring the Charms of Recursion." In *Searching for a Rose Garden: Challenging Psychiatry, Fostering Mad Studies*, edited by Jasna Russo and Angela Sweeney, 172–182. Monmouth, UK: PCCS Books.

Lauveng, Arnhild. 2010. *Morgen bin ich ein Löwe: wie ich die Schizophrenie besiegte*. München: btb.

LeFrançois, Brenda A., Robert Menzies, and Geoffrey Reaume, eds. 2013. *Mad Matters: A Critical Reader in Canadian Mad Studies*. Toronto: Canadian Scholars' Press Inc.

Lehmann, Peter, ed. 2013. *Psychopharmaka absetzen: erfolgreiches Absetzen von Neuroleptika, Antidepressiva, Phasenprophylaktika, Ritalin und Tranquilizern*. Berlin: Antipsychiatrieverlag. (4th edition).

Majerus, Benoît. 2016. "Making Sense of the 'Chemical Revolution'. Patients' Voices on the Introduction of Neuroleptics in the 1950s." *Medical History* 60 (1): 54–66.

Miller, Daniel. 2008. *The Comfort of Things*. Cambridge: Polity.

Penney, Darby, and Peter Stastny. 2009. *The Lives They Left behind: Suitcases from a State Hospital Attic*. New York: Bellevue Literary Press.

Penney, Darby, and Laura Prescott. 2016. "The Co-Optation of Survivor Knowledge: The Danger of Substituted Values and Voice." In *Searching for a Rose Garden: Challenging Psychiatry, Fostering Mad Studies*, edited by Jasna Russo and Angela Sweeney, 35–45. PCCS Books.

Reid, Jenna, Sarah N. Snyder, Jijian Voronka, Danielle Landry, and Kathryn Church. 2019. "Mobilizing Mad Art in the Neoliberal University: Resisting Regulatory Efforts by Inscribing Art as Political Practice." *Journal of Literary & Cultural Disability Studies* 13 (3): 255–71.

Reville, David, and Kathryn Church. 2012. "Mad Activism Enters its Fifth Decade: A Snapshot of Psychiatric Survivor Organizing in Toronto." *In Organize! Building from the Local for Global Justice*, edited by Aziz Choudry, Jill Hanley, and Eric Shragge, n.p. Oakland CA: PM Press.

Schmiedebach, Heinz-Peter, ed. 2016. *Entgrenzungen des Wahnsinns: Psychopathie und Psychopathologisierungen um 1900*. Berlin et al.: De Gruyter.

Schröttle, Monika. 2015. "Lebenssituation und Gewalterfahrungen von Frauen mit sogenannter geistiger Behinderung." In *Sexuell traumatisierte Menschen mit geistiger Behinderung: Forschung – Prävention – Hilfen*, edited by Ulrike Mattke, 29–39. Stuttgart: Kohlhammer.

Schulz, Gwen. 2011. "Spuren-Suche. Zu-Trauen, Geduld, Übersetzen, Hoffen – mein Wunsch an Psychotherapie." In *Psychosenpsychotherapie im Dialog: zur Gründung des DDPP*, edited by Dorothea von Haebler et al, 116–123. Göttingen: Vandenhoeck & Ruprecht.

Sweeney, Angela, ed. 2009. *This Is Survivor Research*. Ross-on-Wye: PCCS Books.

Voronka, Jijian. 2004. *The Race to Space Madness: Making Respectability through Mad Sites in Ontario*. Ottawa: National Library of Canada = Bibliothèque nationale du Canada.

Voronka, Jijian. 2019. "Storytelling Beyond the Psychiatric Gaze: Resisting Resilience and Recovery Narratives." *Canadian Journal of Disability Studies* 8 (4): 8–30.

Wallcraft, J., J. Read, and A. Sweeney. 2003. "On our Own Terms: Users and Survivors of Mental Health Services Working Together for Support and Change." *Sainsbury: Centre for Mental Health*.

Willig, Carla. 2017. "Reflections on the Use of Object Elicitation." *Qualitative Psychology* 4 (3): 211–22.

CHAPTER 11

"There Was an Awful Lot that Was Good and that Was Necessary": the Hidden Heritage of the Old State Mental Hospitals

Verusca Calabria

Abstract

The prevailing perception of the now-closed old state mental hospitals in Britain as outmoded and undesirable has obscured the emotional connections that some former patients and retired staff have for these sites. It has had the effect of effacing the personal histories of mental health service users and workers who hold positive memories of the care provided therein. Drawing on oral histories of former patients and retired staff and community collections of hospital artefacts, this chapter aims to explore the implications of the enforced amnesia of meaningful care practices in the old system for the historiography and heritage of now-defunct psychiatric institutions. It exposes the often-unexplored impacts of deinstitutionalization and the failures of care in community.

Keywords

Deinstitutionalization – enforced amnesia – Ervin Goffman – hidden heritage – oral history

1   Introduction

Since the 1960s, asylums have been presented as sites of incarceration and patient abuse. Ervin Goffman's influential theory (1961) on the nature of closed institutions with their main purpose resting on the close control of the residents, leading to depersonalization, had a profound impact on delegitimising institutional psychiatry (Scull 2010), as did the social movements concerned with exposing the paternalism of coercive psychiatry in favour of liberty and autonomy (Crossley 2006). A point not usually highlighted about psychiatric institutions is their role as places of safety and sanctuary, of patients liking life in hospital and their regrets about its demise (see Gittins 1998; Calabria 2016). These counter representations have not usually been told in published accounts because they do not easily fit within the prevailing discourse of residential care as undesirable and with government policies on deinstitutionalization (Calabria, Bailey, and Bowpitt 2021). In addition, the over-emphasis on the dehumanising and depersonalising institutional practices of psychiatry's past tends to obscure oppressive practices in the current mental health system (Punzi 2019). The dominant perception of the now defunct state mental hospitals as 'total institutions' in the UK and elsewhere has had the effect of erasing knowledge of the positive therapeutic elements of residential care that existed therein.

Patient experiences of care in institutions continue to remain an unexplored area of research (Porter 1985; Coleborne 2020). In addition, the perspectives of nurses and non-medical staff on institutional care practices remain marginalised in the history of psychiatry (McCrae and Peter Nolan 2016). In the examinations of museums and their narratives, the studies of the histories of mental health and institutions have been overlooked in the context of heritage and museum interpretation (Ellis 2015), with a few exceptions such as the work of Coleborne and MacKinnon (2012) on the cultural heritage of psychiatric asylums in Australia and the more recent volume on the material cultures of psychiatry by Ankele and Majerus (2021). Former psychiatric asylum sites are containers of memory for those who lived and worked in them; real estate developers have been operating a form of 'strategic forgetting' of the old asylum buildings. Most of the redevelopment brochures and planning documents have removed its history, thus operating a form of selective remembrance to remove the stigma attached to their bricks and mortar (Kearns, Joseph, and Moon 2010). The main issue with memorialising the old Victorian asylum buildings rests on their contested histories (see, for example, Moon, and Kearns 2016; Gibbeson 2018).

The aim of this chapter is to expose the lack of a unified narrative in relation to the legacy of mental hospitals. In order to pursue this argument, I consider the impact of forcefully silencing positive historical experiences of inpatient care that do not easily fit within the prevailing discourse of residential care as undesirable, and the implications of this enforced amnesia for historiography and heritage of psychiatric institutions. The chapter aims to add to recent academic and community based public history and heritage initiatives which have engaged with the social and cultural history of former psychiatric hospitals across England, Scotland and Wales by highlighting the contested histories of psychiatry, institutions and mental health care.[1] The chapter draws on two collaboratively produced heritage of mental healthcare projects: (1) The oral testimonies of ex-patients and former staff of two now-closed state mental hospitals in Nottinghamshire, UK, collected 30 years after their closure (Calabria 2021); (2) A subsequent oral history project which documented the hidden heritage of local mental healthcare provision, culminating in a co-produced online exhibition.[2]

2   The Projects

My doctoral study, *The Oral Histories of the Nottinghamshire Mental Hospitals*, focused on the lived experiences of mental health service users and professionals who gave and received care in the now-closed Mapperley and Saxondale mental hospitals in Nottinghamshire (UK) across a period of 50 years (Calabria 2020). Mapperley hospital, originally the Borough of Nottingham Lunatic Asylum, opened in 1880 and closed in 1994. Saxondale hospital opened in 1902 as the Radcliffe County Asylum to replace the Sneinton Lunatic Asylum, which was demolished; the hospital closed its doors in 1988. The study explored what may have been lost with the modernisation of mental health services, in the context of the fragmentation of contemporary services, which tend to veer towards crisis management. Twenty people with first-hand experience of giving and receiving care were interviewed multiple times. These included six former patients and fourteen retired medical and non-medical staff who gave and received care at the hospitals between 1948 and 1994. There has been a long-established tradition of innovation in mental health services in Nottingham, such as the introduction of early community care, therapeutic community principles and open-door policy from the 1940s onwards (see, for example, Macmillan 1958; Ramon 2018).

I employed participatory action research (PAR) as an overall framework, and oral history as a data collection strategy, which are both interpretative and grounded mainly in the lived experiences of individuals (Calabria and Bailey 2023). PAR invites participants to become active in all aspects of the research cycle; it differs from other approaches to health and social care research as it seeks the active involvement of stakeholders with the aim of improving care

---

1   See, for example, Whittingham Lives project. Available at: https://whittinghamlives.org.uk/ (accessed September 20, 2022).
2   Hidden Memories of Nottingham Mental Healthcare. Available at: https://www.mental healthcarememories.co.uk/ (accessed March 10, 2021).

and reducing inequalities.[3] Oral history was employed to uncover how former patients, whose historical experiences remain widely marginalised, experienced the closure of the mental hospitals, and to shed light on the complex meanings of care practices therein. The choice of employing oral history was influenced by my long-standing practice as a community-based oral historian, prior to pursuing a career in academia. I embrace a socialist approach to oral history in order to give legitimacy and value to histories from below by amplifying the voices of those who are usually excluded from the public discourse. Oral history is the recording, preservation and interpretation of first-hand accounts of the past (Perks and Thomson 2015). It has often been associated with both grassroots and progressive politics, the democratic desire to amplify the voices of marginalised and oppressed groups (Thompson 2017). The method can give those who are less socially powerful a central place in the creation of their own histories. Oral history holds the potential to balance the documentary evidence, which tells us very little about the patient's experience and even less about the interactions between patients and staff (Calabria, Bailey, and Bowpitt 2021, 195). The main aim of combining these two methodologies was to facilitate the active participation of research subjects, who usually occupy a passive role in traditional research. The study relied on a mix of one-to-one and group encounters to build a shared understanding of how the research would take place, what kind of data would be collected and how meanings would be derived from the data and used to generate findings, including a shared plan for dissemination. Some of the ex-patients' family members and carers took part in group discussions to aid planning of the project and reflection on the findings as they emerged.

Participants' co-produced testimonies about life in the psychiatric hospitals from the mid-twentieth century onwards reveal these institutions to be much more than just entities of social control, instead also being significant spaces laden with meanings that go beyond their purpose as psychiatric care spaces but as relational healthcare systems, the testimonies echo findings from Parr, Philo and Burns' empirical study (2003) in relation to the meanings that patients and staff attached to Craig Dunain Hospital, Scotland, after its closure in 2000. The oral testimonies collected as part of this participatory-driven oral history study challenged the historical position of psychiatric hospitals as institutions solely associated with the misuse of power by providing a reappraisal of the value of inpatient mental health care. The research identified hidden positives of British institutional spaces for service users, perceived to

---

3 It is part of a growing trend of action-oriented research in health and social care for its empowering and inclusive features (see Ward, and Bailey 2011).

be lost in current settings, shedding light on the impacts of deinstitutionalization across a range of policy landscapes, disciplines and settings (Calabria 2022b). The emergent themes from the oral testimonies reveal the symbolic and emotional meanings evoked through the practices of giving and receiving care such as family-like environments, the concepts of home and belonging, remembered as being central to recovery. It demonstrates the paramount importance of the therapeutic environment of the mental hospital and the relationships fostered therein for service users' recovery (Calabria, Bailey, and Bowpitt 2021). The findings capture the loss of the hospital communities as places of safety and belonging and a loss of heritage from the now closed and/ or demolished institutions (Calabria 2022b).

As part of the PAR cycles of reflection, the group meetings encouraged ownership and collective action for both former patients and retired staff, some of whom were carers. Examples include participants formulating a collective plan for dissemination (Calabria and Bailey 2023, 673) of the findings through talks aimed at key decision makers in the community and the public at large to make visible the legacy of meaningful care practices in the now-closed psychiatric institutions. Many felt a deep sense of loss caused by the removal of the signs of the hospitals' history by developers and wanted to preserve and share the hospitals' social history. Former patients set up a group to research the history of a local psychiatric day hospital, reminiscent of other former hospital communities that have established groups to share their own histories (see, for example, Osbourne 2003). Former patients shared their transcripts with others to increase awareness of the importance of having access to a welcoming environment during crisis. In this respect, participants' reciprocal relationships with each other demonstrated overtures of survivor-controlled research, which by its very nature sets off a collective process that instigates ownership of the research (Russo 2012).

Former patients and retired staff suggested more actions to bring about practical change, expressing a need to explore and document the hidden heritage of early community care in Nottingham following the National Health Service and Community Care Act of 1990. To this end, external funding was secured for the co-production of an exhibition in 2020, which led to the second project "Hidden Memories of Nottingham Mental Healthcare."[4] The project was meant to be developed collaboratively with former staff and patients of the Nottingham mental hospitals as well as their families, friends and allies, who remembered the closures and the move to care in the community in the

---

4 Hidden Memories of Nottingham Mental Healthcare. Available at https://www.mental healthcarememories.co.uk/ (accessed March 10, 2021).

1990s. The project was originally envisioned to record and reflect on participants personal and collective community strengths and concerns in relation
to mental well-being, promote dialogue and knowledge exchange among communities of interest and the wider public. Working in partnership with Middle
Street Resource Centre,[5] Rushcliffe Mental Health Carers and the Nottinghamshire Healthcare Foundation Trust, the project was meant to deliver a series of
public Down Memory Lane events to invite participants to reminisce about the
changing experiences of mental health care during the transition from institutional to community care, supported by archival research, including training
on how to access historical archives and digital photography to document local
places that represent individual and collective experiences of mental health
care. The reminiscences, alongside the historical artefacts and digital photographs, were to inform the co-production of a touring exhibition. However, due
to the COVID-19 pandemic and successive lockdowns, the project was reconceptualised into a remote oral history project. Five student placements were
created to help record the memories of stakeholders remotely; myself and the
students collected a total of seventeen oral histories. Nine former nurses, five
social workers, two carers and one local health authority officer who remembered the transition to community care came forward and were interviewed
(Calabria 2022b).

Although there had been initial enthusiasm for the project, we were unable
to reach out to service users who remembered the transition from institutional
to community care provision as Middle Street Resource centre shut due to
COVID-19; no one responded to our online promotion campaign. Access to the
local archives was not possible due to COVID-19 either. Instead, with the help
of participants, a discrete community collection of personal photographs and
memorabilia was gathered, which went to inform a digital audio-visual exhibition. Although co-production was difficult to achieve under the circumstances,
a level of decision-sharing was possible through returning the transcripts
to participants and asking individuals to help choose which textual/audio
extracts and images to put on display to best represent their experiences. The
exhibition was organised along three main themes, namely care in the mental
hospital, transition to community care and experiences of early care in the

---

5   Middle Street Resource Centre is a service user-led organization with a long history of co-
    production. Rushcliffe Mental Health Carers is a self-help group which has been providing
    advice and support to mental health carers in Nottingham, UK, for 25 years; the Nottingham-
    shire Healthcare Foundation Trust is responsible for the provision of mental health services
    in the county of Nottinghamshire, UK.

community.[6] Multiple perspectives about the changing dimension of the provision of care emerged; however, what was common across all the interviews
was a sense of the loss of the hospital communities as places of belonging and
the loss of a place of safety. Although all who were involved in the set-up of
community care were positive about the move to treat people with long-term
mental health needs in the community, what emerged was an ambivalence
about the new system, lacking the warmth and the familiar relationships that
were remembered to be part of the old system. This is concomitant with what
former patients felt about the care provided in the old state mental hospitals
in Nottingham, when compared to their experiences of inpatient care in acute
units as part of the new system (Calabria 2022a). All bemoaned the loss of
investment in mental health care services since the early years of community
care. The oral histories from these projects raise important implications about
the hospitals' remembrance, 30 years since their closure, in light of the failings
of care in the community for those in need of safe spaces when undergoing
crisis and convalescence. As Punzi and Lindbom argue in this volume, narrating the multiple and complex lived experiences of psychiatric care in the
twentieth century and beyond are central to understanding the heritage of
psychiatry.

3   Destruction of Sites of Memory

The oral histories of ex-patients and of retired staff, recorded as part of the first
study, convey an overwhelming sense of nostalgia for the old system of care,
reminiscent of other oral histories of life in mental hospitals in the mid-to-
late twentieth century (Calabria 2022c). As part of a group gathering to discuss
the impact of the study, all expressed finding comfort in the process of reflecting on their historical experiences of receiving care therein. Former patients
felt silenced by their inability to talk about their time at the hospital due to
the stigma attached to having been a patient, as well as the stigma attached to
the asylum sites. They also expressed sadness about the absence of the explicit
memorialisation of the old state mental hospitals. In this sense, the oral history method had the inherent capacity to empower narrators through the process of the telling (Thompson 2017). Kay, for instance, experienced a mental
breakdown in 1991, which led her to attempt suicide. She was subsequently
admitted to Mapperley hospital for a period of 5 months. In her oral testimony,

6   Link to the audio-visual exhibition: https://www.mentalhealthcarememories.co.uk/audio
    -visual-exhibition (accessed March 11, 2021).

Kay stressed the importance of having access to a safe environment that the hospital provided during her mental health crisis:

> There was an awful lot that was good and that was necessary, care in the community often doesn't work because the community is where everything goes wrong, what Mapperley hospital did for me was relieve the situation that had caused me to have a breakdown, I needed to be taken out of the situation, because I was on this treadmill that was going too fast for me, and I'd have had to stay on it if I hadn't been taken out of circulation for a while.

For Kay, the closure of the hospital was misjudged, associating deinstitutionalization with a form of robbery:

> Unfortunately we lost the baby with the bathwater with blowing these institutions away, the propaganda that was put around about these buildings was that they were old Victorian institutions, it might have been true that they were difficult economically to match modern building and facilities but in actual fact they had moved with the times like any other institutions and they were much more progressive than anybody was prepared to concede, mentally ill people were being robbed of the facilities that they had.

Albert, another ex-patient, had repeated hospitalisations at Mapperley hospital for his anxiety disorder (1971, 1981, 1990). He took part in group therapy, describing the sessions as helpful to his recovery, such as learning coping techniques from other patients. He set up his own anxiety self-help group in the community as a result of the help he got from the hospital's therapy group. Albert had fond memories of the care he received at the hospital, recalling that "Mapperley hospital did wonders for me, all in all I can't complain that I as an individual at 80 years of age, that I've not had the attention". Albert recounted very negative experiences of care in the acute wards of the general hospital, which replaced Mapperley hospital in the mid-1990s, he felt that were not suitable to care for people with mental ill health: "I'm glad for everybody's sake that they closed the psychiatric wards there [at the general hospital] because they were not wards in my opinion suitable for mental patients". He recalled that Mapperley hospital was a much more caring and supportive environment than the acute units at the general hospital. He reflected on the importance of accessing a place of refuge during his recurrent mental health crises, recounting that "when you lose the sense of who you are, the importance of feeling safe and protected is more important than anything else". He regretted that younger service users are not able to gain access to the care provided in the old system:

> The younger people that were in for like depression or anxiety, they would keep coming back, I think they would have found that a bit difficult, because they knew that if they were feeling poorly again and then they needed to come into hospital, they knew that they were coming back to Mapperley where people cared for them, people knew them, and then all of a sudden it was taken away from them.

Albert remained incapacitated by his mental health condition and was unable to work for most of his life. A staff member at Mapperley hospital he became friends with encouraged him to volunteer at the hospital. He volunteered as a minibus driver for eight years, which he thoroughly enjoyed. He felt that the legacy of Mapperley hospital was the provision of care for every aspect of a person's needs and felt strongly about preserving its heritage so that the good care that went on in the old system is not forgotten.

Long-serving staff who worked at the Nottingham mental hospitals until their closure brought along ephemera, such as photographs of everyday hospital immaterial culture and official hospital documents that were rescued after the local hospitals closed. These 'documents of life' complemented the process of researching participants' life experiences, not only as memory probes but also to unravel particular meanings of events and relationships embedded in them (Plummer 2001). These artefacts helped to reassert former staff's sense of belonging to the hospital communities. All recounted witnessing the removal of the hospitals' material culture. They saw historical documentation being thrown into skips while the hospital was emptied, which they then rescued in an effort to retain the memory of the hospital.

Craig was born at Saxondale hospital in 1959 and grew up on site; both his parents worked as nurses and lived at the hospital until their deaths. He became a porter and worked on site until it closed in 1988, transferring to work as an electrician at Mapperley hospital. He was keen to emphasise that the strict hierarchy between medical and non-medical staff relaxed significantly in the 1970s as part of the shift in focus towards the social rehabilitation of patients. He explained that he lived at the hospital during "the heyday period" when the social model of mental health was embraced. He remembered that the relationships that were formed between the general staff and the patients were genuine friendships which had been fostered through living on the site of the hospital as part of a community: "the patients accepted me as part of the community because they knew me as a child, they would be quite open with me, they would come to see us the porters, sit down and gossip". Craig turned up for his first oral history interview with a bundle of historical documents he rescued. These included life documents, such as a photograph of the Saxondale football club. He recalled that "I was one of those who bundled up pictures and documents for safekeeping as Saxondale closed. I found a few documents in the skip when Mapperley subsequently closed". He talked about the importance of the football team for engendering a sense of pride within the hospital community: "In my father's day, one of the things they were proud of was the staff won cups because it shone some glory on the hospital and it provided entertainment for the patients".

Louise came over to England from the Caribbean in 1978 and went to work as a nurse at Saxondale hospital until its closure in 1988. She still lives in the original tied house the hospital provided. She recalled that Saxondale was a "heaven" for both the patients and the staff:

> Some patients had lived there from when they were very young so it was home for them and although they used to get a lot of visitors from their families, only some because a lot of them were just forgotten, what staff would ensure is that they were treated like family.

For Louise, the community that existed therein, made up of three generations of medical and non-medical staff, provided a rich source of social support for residents. When the hospital closed, the loss of a sense of community caused social isolation for people with enduring mental ill health. She recalled that "things are different now, they've lost what was their community, many of the people that were pushed out became socially isolated, there were not enough community services to compensate".

Louise felt that "care in the community is awful" as the patients had lost the ability to walk around and out of the hospital on their own and lost access to outdoor spaces; she stressed the return to institutional practices of pre-open door policy in the current system limited the choice for clients; she felt that it would have been preferable to improve the old system rather than start a completely new provision of care:

> Quite frankly I am not keen with care in the community, if the improvement in the new places could have been done in the large psychiatric hospitals with all that was there, I think that would have been better. Where people used to have really severe mental health problems, you used to have space to explore, now they are locked into a limited space

in psychiatric units in general hospitals, that sense of freedom and that sense of healing environment and atmosphere isn't out there.

During her first oral history interview, Louise brought three folders of documents pertaining to the preparations the hospital made to support long-stay patients to move out into the community, which she rescued when the hospital closed. She was upset that the efforts that staff made at the time to support the transition to community care had been erased with the dumping of these documents. The act of rescuing these documents poses the important question about how the material culture relating to institutions can be used to provide more representative histories of psychiatry's past. Ellis argues that the medical profession wanted to save mental hospital records for preservation and reuse in museum settings in order to particularly tell the positive and progressive history of mental health care at a time when institutional care was being critiqued (Ellis 2015). However, Craig and Louise rescued and personally preserved both official and life documents relating to the life of Saxondale hospital as a form of resistance against the erasure of the rich social history of the hospital communities and their impetus to preserve its legacy from oblivion. In addition, Craig felt insulted by the estate developers who changed the names of the streets to erase the official memory of the hospital. He explained how local residents tried to resist the changes and were able to retain the name 'Saxondale' for the main drive leading up to the estate while dropping the word 'hospital'. For Craig, the government and the developers "eradicated the history of the hospital", providing evidence of the forced amnesia of mental hospitals as deeply stigmatised sites (Kearns, Alun, and Moon 2010). In his oral history testimony, he compared the closure and subsequent erasure of its history to the destruction of a village during wartime:

> It's like a war destroyed my village because the village is gone, they split everyone up, the people you work with are gone, the patients you talked to are gone, the memories [...] the signs have gone, and everything is called something different now.

Roger grew up on the Saxondale hospital site in the 1950s, his father was a nurse; he worked as an electrician until the hospital closed in the mid-1980s. Although he experienced stigma as a child in school because he lived at Saxondale, he had very fond memories of life at the hospital. He repeatedly referred to the hospital as village-like, he felt proud of the community that existed on site; he knew all the staff as he dealt with every ward as part of his job maintaining the site. For Roger, the impact of closing the hospitals resulted in the loss of kinship between staff and patients. He recalled the familiar relationships fostered between non-medical staff and patients:

> There was a huge amount of domestic staff in those days, they were terrific with the patients, they'd make tea and do lots of other little things that perhaps you wouldn't have to do, alter clothes, all manner of stuff, some of the more touching things I saw, people that were in their last days being nursed.

Roger visited the hospital site after its closure, which was not redeveloped for a number of years: "People had been in and stolen things so it was like watching your village being destroyed, it was awful". He expressed sadness for the lack of care of the abandoned site: "I watched that little village going from being immaculately presented and looked after, people were proud; by the time it closed, no one cared".

Through group discussions with ex-patients and retired staff, a collective consensus emerged about the need to preserve, celebrate and share with a wider audience the intangible heritage of the local mental hospitals. As a result, former patients and retired staff asked to develop the findings of the study into an exhibition about the legacy of the local mental hospitals.[7] Due to COVID-19, the exhibition was curated entirely remotely, including the collection of oral histories and personal artefacts. What follows are some extracts from the interviews that reflect on the hidden legacy of the Nottinghamshire mental hospitals in terms of the loss of the helpful care practices therein.

Joe trained as a social worker in the 1980s. He joined the community team as part of the Rehabilitation and Community Care Service (RSSC) at Nottingham Health Authority in the mid-1980s at a time of innovation. The new multidisciplinary service was responsible for closing down the mental hospitals and rehabilitate 300 to 500 people in the community. Every service user had their own linked worker long-term, either a social worker, a community psychiatric nurse or an occupational therapist in the community. The service bridged the long-stay wards and community care provision, so all staff knew what was available in the community and the risks associated with moving long-stay patients out of the hospital. Joe felt that the mental hospital provided a safe and comfortable environment. At the time of closure, he was concerned about the difficulties of accessing a lot of services available in the institutions that

---

7 The National Lottery Heritage Fund awarded the project a grant in January 2020 to coproduce a permanent exhibition of the intangible heritage of Nottingham Mental Health Provision: https://www.mentalhealthcarememories.co.uk/.

were not easy to access when living in the community. He reflected on what has been lost since the closure of the mental hospitals:

> The asylum offers an all-encompassing organisation for the patient so social and recreational activity, industrial therapy activity, outings, a lot of personal attention to what you need for yourself, for example, hairdressing and chiropody were provided on site. There was weekly physiotherapy on offer for people who had associated physical disabilities along with mental health difficulties, all provided by the service free of charge. That was not going to be the case to that extent when living in a resident home or in a flat. The people in their 60s and 70s who learned to live this way, this was their life. In a way, it would have been far preferable if they just stayed where they were and just that to allow to carry on living in that way whilst people who had repeated admissions to hospital who were much younger would not tolerate that lifestyle, even though it was comfortable.

Joe bemoaned the gradual cuts to mental health budgets and the steady reduction of well-resourced community services in the last 20 years that could offer a high degree of supervision and protection by health hostel provision, which has disappeared. He regretted that no records had been kept of the move from institutional to community-based services:

> This project has made me realise how much work, effort and relationship building went into this whole process. And it's gone. It's a regret that we didn't feel able or didn't feel we needed to or had the time to keep some kind of comprehensive record of what we were doing over those years. We didn't really sit down and say, can we evaluate the impact this has had on the residents or the service users who are now living on somewhere on this continuum range. What's happened to them? And what did they think about what we did?

Judith trained as a psychiatric nurse in 1966 at Mapperley hospital and later joined the School of Nursing at the hospital until she retired in 2006. She worked as a nurse at the Robin Hood ward in the 1970s where group therapy was part of the daily routine of care. She explained her reasons for wanting to preserve the memories of the care provided in the old system and the transition to community care:

> We need a sense of identity of who we are and where we've come from. It's a bit like why we celebrate all the people who fought in the world

wars, so that we don't forget what they did so that we could be as we are today. I think to improve services and treatments and so to look back and think what worked, what didn't work, to carry forward improvements, to remember the kind of legacy that we've left really and not to forget all those people who worked and lived and were patients in those times. It is about keeping it alive so that we can examine our heritage to understand how we've arrived here today, where we've come from and our sense of identity of who we are.

The extracts from these collaboratively produced oral histories with former patients and staff about care practices in psychiatric hospitals in the latter part of the twentieth century reveal these institutions to be meaningful social spaces loaded with significance. The everyday care practices within, viewed through the use of internal and external spaces, could act as a therapeutic landscape. In addition, the oral testimonies are laced with nostalgia, providing evidence of the loss of the hospital communities as places of safety and belonging, and a loss of heritage from the now-closed and/or repurposed institutions (Calabria 2022c). In the case of deinstitutionalization, nostalgia for the old system of care rests in its relationship to present concerns, providing clues to the role it plays in reconstructing identity, as Bennett (2009) has asserted. Nostalgic narratives of institutional care can shed light on how the transferral of care from asylum to community was lived by key actors and how the reconfiguration of care may have affected the capacity for lived experiences of care to be retained and commemorated. Narratives of community decline can serve as a means of registering and understanding dramatic change, helping to preserve a sense of place at a time when collective memories are threatened by the destruction and remaking of urban environments (Ramsden 2016). Repurposing the old county asylums in the UK has materially effaced the memories of place held by those who lived and worked in them.

The oral testimonies of ex-patients and retired staff evidence how these stakeholders are "neither powerless nor fully dominated by external forces, but active participants 'in the cultural negotiations of their identities" (Thompson 1963, 9) in the context of their experiences of hospital care environments. These perspectives open up possibilities for alternative modes of collective remembering and memorialising the 'uncomfortable heritage' of asylums (Pendlebury, Wang, and Law, 2018). The perceived 'threat to heritage' expressed by ex-patients and retired staff raises the question of what constitutes the preservation of heritage in the context of mental health provision, where some stakeholders seek to change perceptions about the past to help shed light on issues faced in the present. The explicit absence of memorialisation of the old system of institutional care are as a direct consequence of the pervasive and sustained collective amnesia of these sites has a direct bearing on erasing individual and collective remembrance of the lived experiences of care practices therein. The emotional attachment to these sites by the communities once contained within them has implications for the preservation of their material and immaterial heritage, calling for its reconceptualization. Participatory-driven oral history work can play a crucial role in redressing the pervasive notion that progress is an inherent feature of mental health policy by gathering eye witness testimonies with communities whose experiences of the changing dimension of care across time have yet to be fully heard. Bosworth defined this kind of research as 'heritage without walls' when facilitating memory work in the contested spaces of Western Australia, where competing versions of the past are held by state authorities and local communities (Bosworth 2013). Fostering the co-production of eye witness testimonies in communities whose stories have not yet become part of the mainstream historical record can become a vehicle for the development of alternative interpretations of the past by under-represented groups. These alternative representations in turn can become part of the collective record (Dodd 2013). Importantly, these oral testimonies help to explore the past of institutional psychiatry to better understand the present of mental health care and community understandings, dispositions, and responses to mental health and the mentally distressed, and enable critical imaginings of better futures.

4   Conclusion

The oral testimonies of former patients and retired staff about life in the old state mental hospitals in the UK in the second half of the twentieth century reveal these environments to be much more permeable than reported in the literature, as Baur has shown in this volume. These memories offer the possibility of remembering the material and immaterial aspects of the local mental hospitals in new and unexpected ways that challenge the forced amnesia about the social life of institutions. The inclusion of the lived experiences of previously neglected key actors, such as non-medical staff, helps to more widely represent life in the mental hospitals in the latter part of the twentieth century. The findings evidence the need for a re-appraisal of the value of care provided in the old state mental hospitals as articulated in the oral testimonies of people who gave and received care therein that bear not only on current mental health policy and practice but on memory work in the context of heritage. The co-produced oral histories demonstrate the value of the immaterial heritage of psychiatry through an exploration of the care practices, such as informal care provided by communities and networks that existed therein. It sheds light on the impact of the destruction of a site of memory in terms of the forced amnesia of mental hospitals as places of belonging. This has given rise to a hidden collective sense of loss, both in terms of access to adequate care, and the inability to remember the old system of care individually and collectively in the present.

Participatory-informed oral history is particularly suitable to explore and document the histories of mental health care and institutions, largely overlooked in the context of the cultural heritage of psychiatry. Participatory methods can offer novel ways of interpreting and memorialising the heritage of psychiatry as Baur has argued in this volume. The oral testimonies of former patients and retired staff discussed in this chapter offer important methodological reflections by examining how the meaning of institutional care differs across time and individual actors and what it tells us about present concerns, in terms of the failure of government to make community care work, with the lack of access to safe spaces during crisis, adding to the widespread criticism of deinstitutionalization and the policy of care in the community, leading to more problems than it solved (Bacopoulos-Viau 2016). One example is re-institutionalisation, where service users who would have been long-term hospitalised before deinstitutionalization are now being transferred to different institutional settings such as residential homes, forensic hospitals and mostly prisons (Chow and Priebe 2013; Kritsotaki, Long, and Smith 2016).

The co-production of exhibitions is becoming an increasingly common method to facilitate public engagement across the medical humanities, which raises its own set of ethical challenges, for which university research ethics boards are not designed to address, as Gagen (2021) has pointed out. One of the main ethical dilemmas arising from my public-engagement research is the tension between uncovering hidden histories that restore agency to silenced actors while also retaining an obligation to sensitively handle individual and collective nostalgic memories of institutional care in order to not cause offence to those who suffered institutional abuse, such as the loss of identity that Lindbom experienced as a result of psychiatric hospitalisation reported in this volume (Punzi & Lindbom, 2023). Another ethical dilemma that can emerge in PAR research is that institutional ethics procedures require researchers to outline the research plan in detail, which is hard to predict in projects of this nature (Bussu and Lalani 2020, 7). Crucially, the contested meanings of care that emerged from these studies offer the opportunity to redress imbalances in the historiography of psychiatry, where certain accounts of the past are held up as being more valid than others (Davies 2001).

As Coleborne (2016) has pointed out, to come closer to a fuller sense of the lived histories of mental health across time, the larger, shared history of psychiatric institutions need to be told to avoid presenting only half a history. Exploring common ground between historians and healthcare professionals by engaging with community-led heritage-based research, such as the 'Heritage and Stigma' project, can help researchers examine not only the role played by memory work in individual and collective histories of mental health but also its implications for inclusive heritage (see Rob Ellis 2017). The 'Hidden Memories of Nottingham Mental Healthcare' project brought to light meaningful aspects of care in the old system overlooked during deinstitutionalization and heralding of community care. Portraying multiple historical experiences of institutional care practices to uncover the intangible heritage of these institutions for diverse stakeholders through the use of applied methodologies requires being open to user-defined paradigm of value. These eye witness accounts help to deepen the focus on the legacies and heritage of psychiatric institutions in the twenty-first century, and their impacts on understanding the current crises in contemporary mental health provision in the UK and elsewhere.

References

Ankele Monika, and Majerus Benoit. 2021. *Material Cultures of Psychiatry*. Bielefeld: Transcript Verlag.

Bacopoulos-Viau, Alexandra. 2016. "The Patient's Turn Roy Porter and Psychiatry's Tales, Thirty Years on." *Medical History* 60, no. 1: 1–18.

Bennett, Katy. 2009. "Telling Tales: Nostalgia, Collective Identity and an Ex-mining Village." In *Emotion, Place and Culture* 8, edited by Mick Smith, Joyce Davidson, and Liz Bondi, 187–206. Abingdon: Routledge.

Bosworth, Michal. 2013. "Let Me Tell You … Memory and the Practice of Oral History." In *Memory and History: Understanding Memory as Source and Subject,* edited by Joan Tumblety, 19–33. Abingdon: Routledge.

Bussu, Sonia, Mirza Lalani, Stephen Pattison, and Martin Marshall. 2020. "Engaging with Care: Ethical Issues in Participatory Research." *Qualitative Research* 25 (5): 1–19. https://doi.org/10.1177/1468794120904883.

Calabria, Verusca. 2016. "Insider Stories from the Asylum: Peer and Staff-Patient Relationships." In *Narrating Illness: Prospects and Constraints,* edited by Joanna Davidson and Yomna Saber, 3–12. Oxford: Interdisciplinary Press.

Calabria, Verusca. 2020. "Oral Histories of the Nottinghamshire Mental Hospitals: Exploring Memories of Giving and Receiving Care." PhD diss. Nottingham Trent University.

Calabria, Verusca. 2023. "An Exploration of the Function of Nostalgia in Oral Histories of Institutional Care." In *Faith in Reform: Anniversaries, Memory and the Asylum in International Historical Perspective*, edited by Rob Ellis, Rebecca Wynter, and Jennifer Wallis, 231–255. Ashgate: Palgrave Macmillan.

Calabria, Verusca. 2022b. "Learning and doing oral History in Higher Education in interdisciplinary contexts in the midst of the COVID-19 pandemic." *Oral History* 50 (2): 107–117.

Calabria, Verusca. 2022a. "With Care in the Community, Everything Goes: Using Oral History to Re-examine the Provision of Care in the Mental Hospitals." *Oral History* 50 (1): 93–103.

Calabria, Verusca, and Di Bailey. 2023. "Participatory Action Research and Oral History as Natural Allies in Mental Health Research." *Qualitative Research* 23 (3): 668–685. https://journals.sagepub.com/doi/10.1177/14687941211039963.

Calabria, Verusca, Di Bailey, and Graham Bowpitt. 2021. "More Than Just Brick and Mortar: Meaningful Care Practices in the Old State Mental Hospitals." In *Voices in the History of Madness: Patient and Practitioner Perspectives*, edited by Rob Ellis, Sarah Kendall, and Steve Taylor, 191–215. Palgrave Macmillan, Mental Health in Historical Perspectives Series.

Chow, Winnie S., Stefan Priebe. 2013. "Understanding Psychiatric Institutionalization: A Conceptual Review." *BMC Psychiatry* 13, no. 1: 1–14.

Coleborne, Catharine, and Dolly MacKinnon. 2012. *Exhibiting Madness in Museums: Remembering Psychiatry Through Collection and Display*, vol. 4. Abingdon: Routledge.

Coleborne, Catharine. 2020. *Why Talk About Madness? Bringing History into the Conversation*. Abingdon: Palgrave Macmillan, Mental Health in Historical Perspectives Series.

Coleborne, Catharine. 2016. "Talk, Dissent, Silence: Narrating Madness in the Twentieth Century." Keynote Address, Voices of Madness Conference, Centre for Health Histories, University of Huddersfield, UK.

Crossley, Nick. 2006. *Contesting Psychiatry: Social Movements in Mental Health*. Abingdon: Routledge.

Davies, Kerry. 2001. "Silent and Censured Travellers? Patients' Narratives and Patients' Voices: Perspectives on the History of Mental Illness since 1948." *Social History of Medicine* 14, no. 2: 267–292.

Dodd, Lindsey. 2013. "Small Fish, Big Pond: Using a Single Oral History Narrative to Reveal Broader Social Change." In *Memory and History: Understanding Memory as Source and Subject*, edited by Joan Tumblety, 34–49. Abingdon: Routledge.

Ellis, Rob. 2015. "Without Decontextualization: the Stanley Royd Museum and the Progressive History of Mental Health Care." History of Psychiatry 26, no. 3: 332–347.

Ellis, Rob. 2017. "Heritage and Stigma. Co-Producing and Communicating the Histories of Mental Health and Learning Disability." *Medical Humanities* 43.2: 92–98.

Gagen, Elizabeth. 2021. "Facing Madness: The Ethics of Exhibiting Sensitive Historical Photographs." *Journal of Historical Geography* 71: 39–50.

Gibbeson, Carolyn. 2018. *"After the Asylum: Place, Value and Heritage in the Redevelopment of Historic Former Asylums."* PhD diss., Newcastle University.

Gittins, Diana. 1998. *Madness in its Place: Narratives of Severalls Hospital, 1913–1997.* London and New York: Routledge.

Kearns, Robin, Joseph Alun E., and Graham Moon. 2010. "Memorialisation and Remembrance: On Strategic Forgetting and the Metamorphosis of Psychiatric Asylums into Sites for Tertiary Educational Provision." *Social & Cultural Geography* 11, no. 8: 731–749.

Kritsotaki, Despo, Vicky Long, and Matt Smith. 2016. "Deinstitutionalisation and After: Post-war Psychiatry in the Western World." Asghate: Palgrave Macmillan.

Macmillan, Duncan. 1958. "Mental Health Services of Nottingham." *International Journal of Social Psychiatry* 4, no. 1: 5–9.

McCrae Niall, and Peter Nolan. 2016. *The Story of Nursing in British Mental Hospitals: Echoes from the Corridors.* London and New York: Routledge.

Moon, Graham, and Robin Kearns. 2016. *The Afterlives of the Psychiatric Asylum Recycling Concepts, Sites and Memories.* Abingdon: Routledge.

Osbourne, Ray. 2003. "Asylums as Cultural heritage: The Challenges of Adaptive Re-use." In *Madness in Australia: Histories, Heritage and the Asylum,* edited by Catharine Coleborne and Dolly Mackinnon, 217–227. St Lucia: University of Queensland Press.

Parr, Hester, Chris Philo, and Nicola Burns. 2003. "That Awful Place Was Home: Reflections on the Contested Meanings of Craig Dunain Asylum." *Scottish Geographical Journal* 119, no. 4: 341–360.

Pendlebury, John, Yi-Wen Wang, and Andrew Law. 2018. "Re-using Uncomfortable Heritage: The Case of the 1933 Building, Shanghai." *International Journal of Heritage Studies* 24, no 3: 211–229.

Perks, Robert, and Alistar Thomson. 2015. *The Oral History Reader.* Abingdon: Routledge.

Plummer, Kenneth. 2001. *Documents of Life 2: An Invitation to a Critical Humanism.* London: Thousand Oaks.

Porter, Roy. 1985. "The Patient's View: Doing Medical History from Below." *Theory and Society* 14, no. 2: 175–198.

Punzi, Elisabeth. 2019. "Ghost Walks or Thoughtful Remembrance. How Should the Heritage of Psychiatry be Approached?" *The Journal of Critical Psychology, Counselling and Psychotherapy* 19, no. 4: 242–251.

Ramon, Shulamit. 2018. *Psychiatry in Britain: Meaning and Policy* 18. Abingdon: Routledge.

Ramsden, Stefan. 2016. "The Community Spirit Was a Wonderful Thing: On Nostalgia and the Politics of Belonging." *Oral History* 44, no. 1: 89–97.

Russo, Jasna. 2012. "Survivor-controlled Research: A New Foundation for Thinking About Psychiatry and Mental Health. *Qualitative Social Research* 13, no. 1: 18–24.

Scull, Andrew. 2010. "Psychiatry and the Social Sciences, 1940–2009." *History of Political Economy* Supplement 42, no. 1: 25–52.

Thompson, EP. 1963. *The Making of the English Working Class.* London: Victor Gollancz Ltd.

Thompson, Paul. 2017. *The Voice of the Past: Oral History.* Oxford: Oxford University Press.

Ward James, and Di Bailey. 2011. "At arms' Length: the Development of a Self-Injury Training Package for Prison Staff Through Service User-Involvement." *The Journal of Mental Health Training, Education and Practice,* 6.4:175–185.

Index